Chapter 6 : Satisfying Dinner Recipes

Chapter 7 : Healthy Snacks for Hormonal Balance

Table of Contents

Chapter 5 : Nutritious Lunch Recipes

Introduction

Menopause is a significant life transition that marks the end of a woman's reproductive years. This natural phase is characterized by hormonal changes, which can bring about a variety of symptoms such as hot flashes, night sweats, mood swings, and weight gain. While menopause is a natural part of aging, its impact on a woman's body can be challenging. One of the most effective ways to manage these changes and promote overall well-being is through nutrition. The right diet can help alleviate symptoms, maintain a healthy weight, and support bone health and mood stability.

The "Menopause Reset Cookbook" is designed to provide women with the knowledge and recipes needed to navigate this phase with confidence and vitality. This cookbook isn't just about recipes; it's about understanding the nutritional needs during menopause and how specific foods can make a significant difference in how you feel. We will explore the essential nutrients that play a crucial role in hormonal balance, energy levels, and overall health.

Each chapter of this cookbook is dedicated to a different aspect of menopause nutrition. From understanding the fundamentals of menopausal nutrition to specific recipes for breakfast, lunch, dinner, snacks, and desserts, you'll find a wealth of information and delicious meals to support your health. Additionally, we will cover plant-based options, weight management strategies, and ways to address common menopausal symptoms through diet.

Chapter 1: Understanding Menopause and Nutrition

Menopause typically occurs between the ages of 45 and 55, although it can start earlier or later. It is defined as the point in time 12 months after a woman's last menstrual period. The years leading up to that point are called perimenopause, during which women may experience various symptoms due to fluctuating hormone levels, particularly estrogen and progesterone.

The relationship between menopause and nutrition is significant. Hormonal changes during menopause can lead to a variety of health issues, including:

- Bone Density Loss: Decreased estrogen levels can lead to bone loss, increasing the risk of osteoporosis.

- Weight Gain: Hormonal shifts can cause weight gain, particularly around the abdomen.

- Heart Health: The risk of cardiovascular disease increases after menopause.

- Mood Swings: Hormonal fluctuations can affect mood and mental health.

- Energy Levels: Many women report feeling fatigued during menopause.

Understanding these changes and how nutrition can help manage them is crucial. A balanced diet rich in essential nutrients can help mitigate these symptoms and support overall health. Key nutrients to focus on during menopause include calcium, vitamin D, magnesium, phytoestrogens, omega-3 fatty acids, and antioxidants.

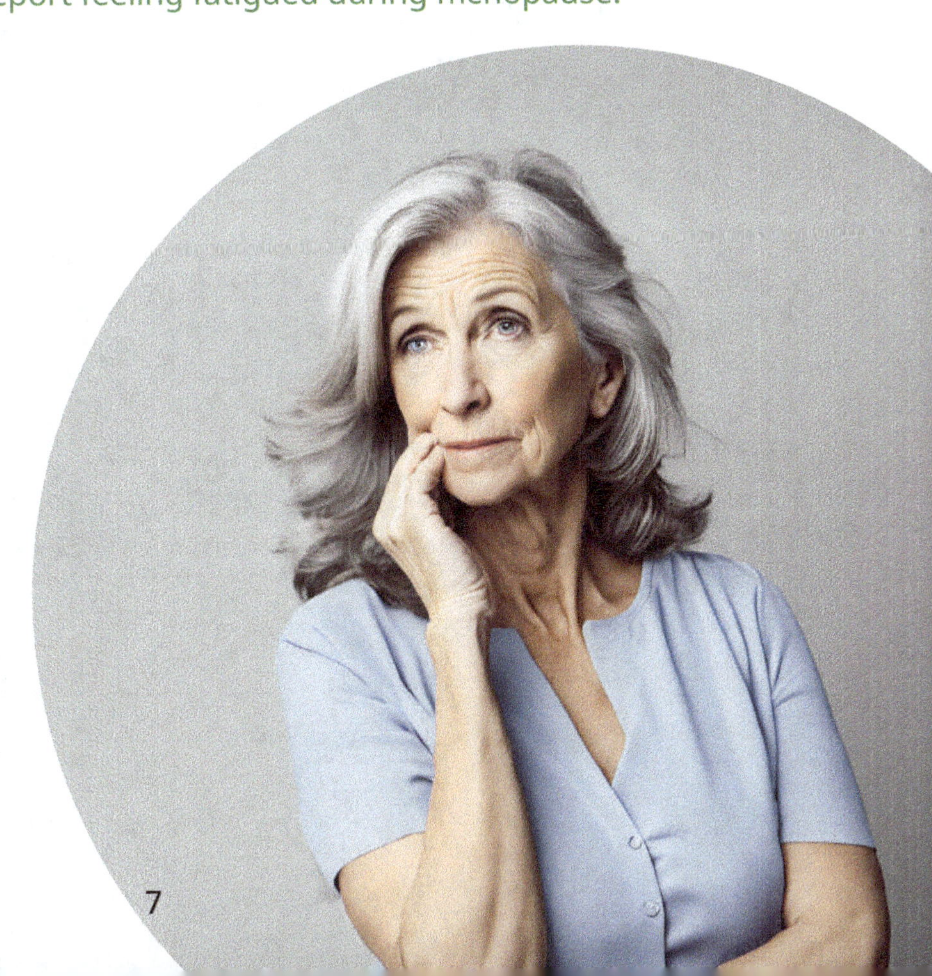

Chapter 2: Essential Nutrients for Menopausal Health

To navigate menopause with grace and health, focusing on essential nutrients is paramount. Here, we delve into the specific nutrients that are particularly beneficial during this stage of life:

- Calcium and Vitamin D: Vital for bone health. Calcium-rich foods include dairy products, leafy greens, and fortified foods. Vitamin D is essential for calcium absorption and can be obtained from sunlight, fatty fish, and fortified foods.

- Magnesium: Supports bone health and reduces the risk of osteoporosis. Magnesium-rich foods include nuts, seeds, legumes, and whole grains.

- Phytoestrogens: Plant-based compounds that mimic estrogen and can help balance hormones. Sources include soy products, flaxseeds, and whole grains.

- Omega-3 Fatty Acids: Essential for heart health and reducing inflammation. Found in fatty fish, flaxseeds, chia seeds, and walnuts.

- Antioxidants: Protect cells from damage and support overall health. Abundant in fruits, vegetables, nuts, and seeds.

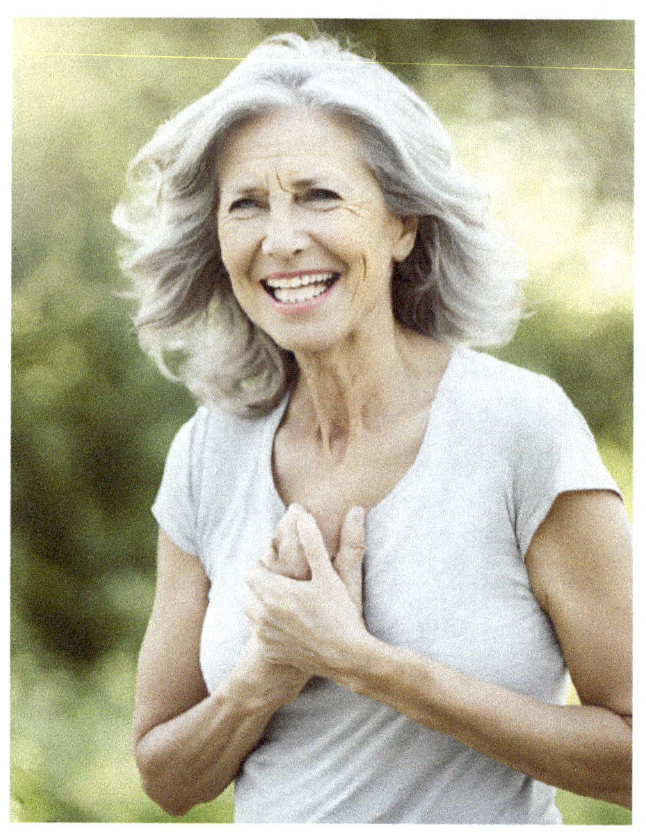

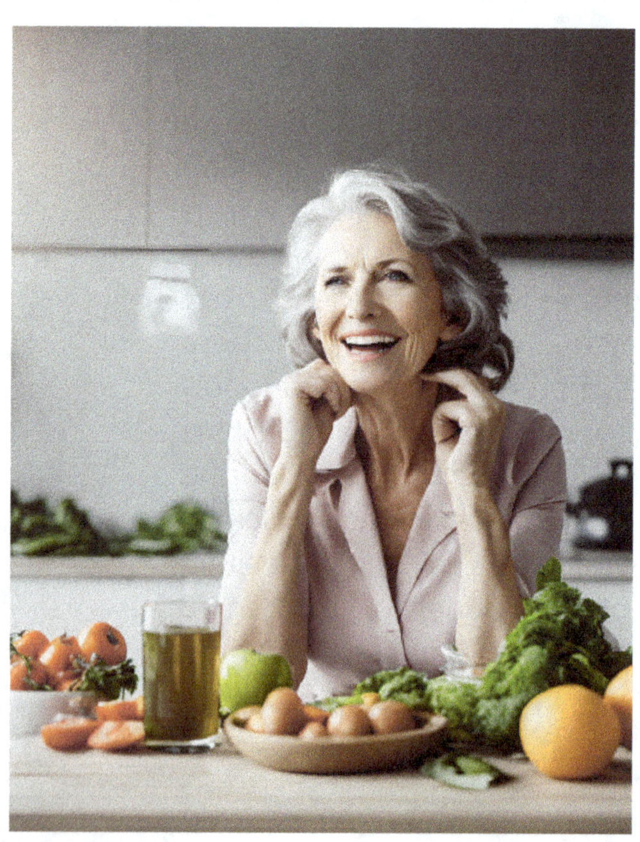

Chapter 3: Building a Balanced Menopause-Friendly Diet

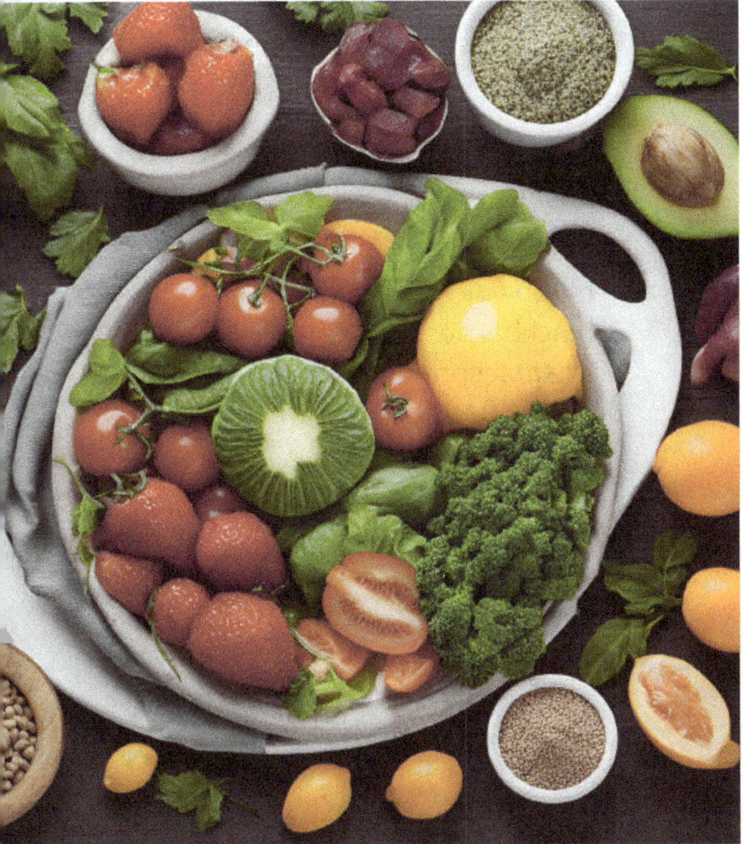

Creating a balanced diet that supports your health during menopause involves incorporating a variety of nutrient-dense foods. Here are some guidelines to help you build a menopause-friendly diet:

- Prioritize Whole Foods: Focus on whole, minimally processed foods such as fruits, vegetables, whole grains, lean proteins, and healthy fats.

- Balance Macronutrients: Ensure a good balance of carbohydrates, proteins, and fats in your meals to maintain energy levels and support overall health.

- Include Phytoestrogens: Incorporate soy products, flaxseeds, and other phytoestrogen-rich foods into your diet to help balance hormones.

- Hydrate: Drink plenty of water to stay hydrated, which is crucial for overall health and well-being.

- Limit Sugar and Refined Carbs: Reduce your intake of sugary foods and refined carbohydrates to help manage weight and blood sugar levels.

- Mind Your Portions: Be mindful of portion sizes to maintain a healthy weight.

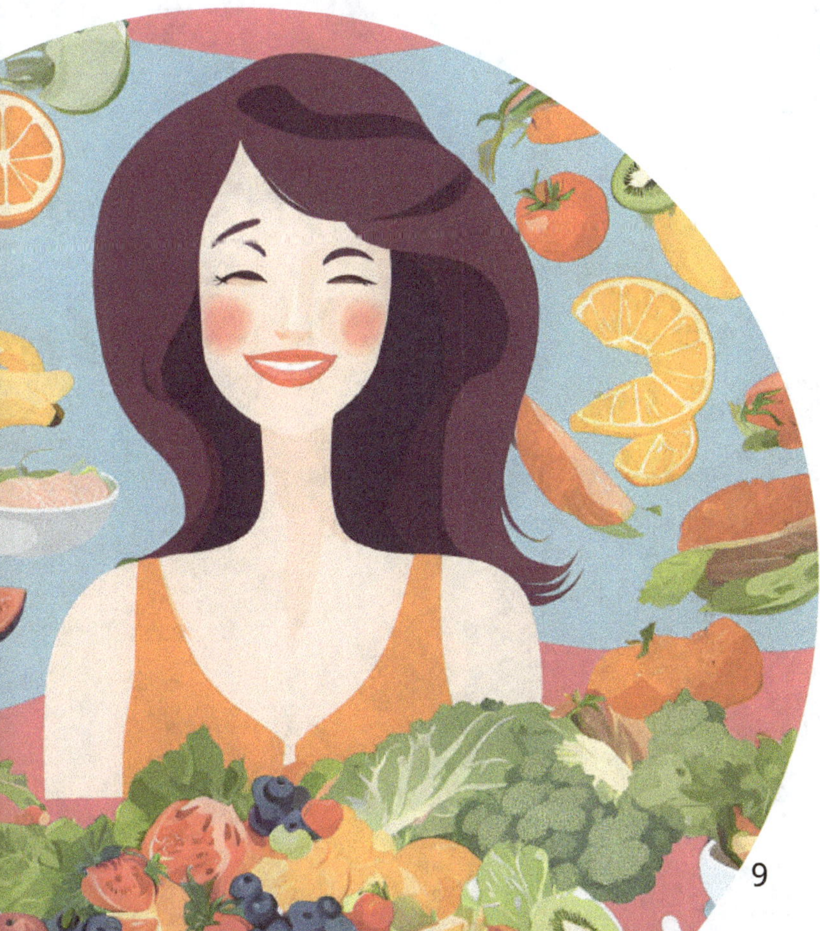

1. Greek Yogurt with Berries and Honey

Preparation Time: 5 minutes
Cook Time: 0 minutes
Total Time: 5 minutes

Serves: 1

Ingredients:

1 cup plain Greek yogurt
- 1/2 cup mixed berries (such as blueberries, raspberries, and/or blackberries)
- 1 tablespoon honey

Directions:

1. Place the Greek yogurt in a serving bowl.

2. Top the yogurt with the mixed berries.

3. Drizzle the honey over the top.

4. Serve immediately.

Nutrition Facts (per serving):
- Calories: 200
- Total Fat: 5g
- Saturated Fat: 3g
- Cholesterol: 15mg
- Sodium: 65mg
- Total Carbohydrates: 23g
- Dietary Fiber: 3g
- Sugars: 19g
- Protein: 17g

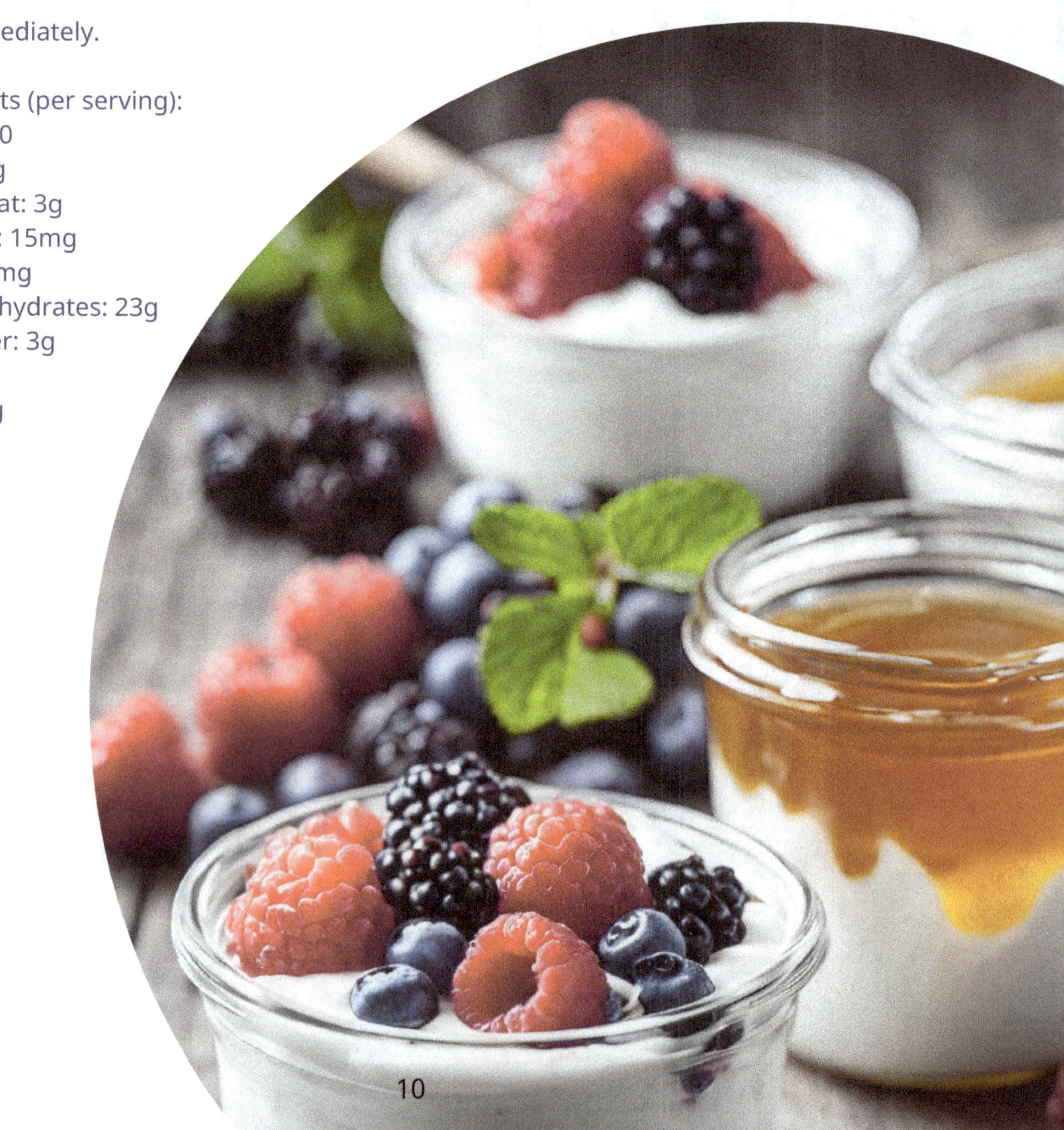

2. Oatmeal with Flaxseeds and Banana

Preparation Time: 5 minutes
Cook Time: 10 minutes
Total Time: 15 minutes

Serves: 1

Ingredients:

 1/2 cup old-fashioned rolled oats
- 1 cup unsweetened almond milk (or milk of your choice)
- 1 tablespoon ground flaxseeds
- 1 ripe banana, sliced
- 1 teaspoon honey (optional)

Directions:

1. In a small saucepan, combine the rolled oats and almond milk.

2. Bring the mixture to a simmer over medium heat, stirring occasionally, until the oats are tender and the milk has thickened, about 8-10 minutes.

3. Remove the oatmeal from the heat and stir in the ground flaxseeds.

4. Transfer the oatmeal to a serving bowl and top with the sliced banana.

5. Drizzle the honey over the top, if desired.

Nutrition Facts (per serving):
- Calories: 320
- Total Fat: 8g
- Saturated Fat: 1g
- Cholesterol: 0mg
- Sodium: 75mg
- Total Carbohydrates: 54g
- Dietary Fiber: 8g
- Sugars: 16g
- Protein: 9g

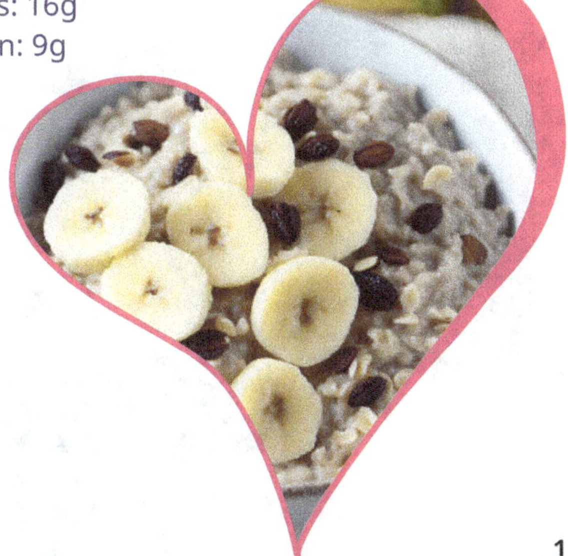

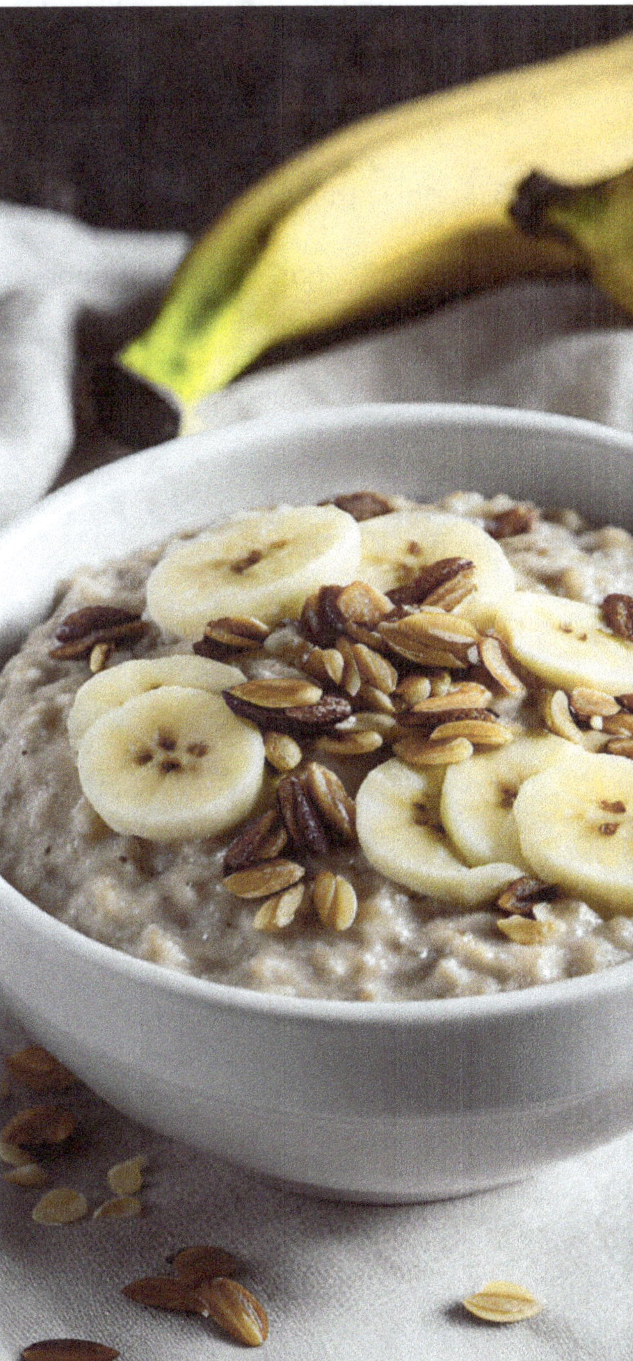

3. Avocado Toast with Whole Grain Bread

Preparation Time: 5 minutes
Cook Time: 0 minutes
Total Time: 5 minutes

Serves: 1

Directions:

1. Toast the whole grain bread until lightly golden.

2. In a small bowl, mash the avocado with a fork.

3. Spread the mashed avocado evenly over the toasted bread slices.

4. Drizzle the olive oil over the avocado toast.

5. Sprinkle the salt and black pepper over the top.

6. If desired, garnish with chopped fresh cilantro or parsley.

Nutrition Facts (per serving, 2 slices):
- Calories: 320
- Total Fat: 20g
- Saturated Fat: 3g
- Cholesterol: 0mg
- Sodium: 460mg
- Total Carbohydrates: 32g
- Dietary Fiber: 9g
- Sugars: 3g
- Protein: 7g

Ingredients:
 2 slices whole grain bread
- 1 ripe avocado, mashed
- 1 tablespoon olive oil
- 1/4 teaspoon salt
- 1/4 teaspoon black pepper
- 1 tablespoon chopped fresh cilantro or parsley (optional)

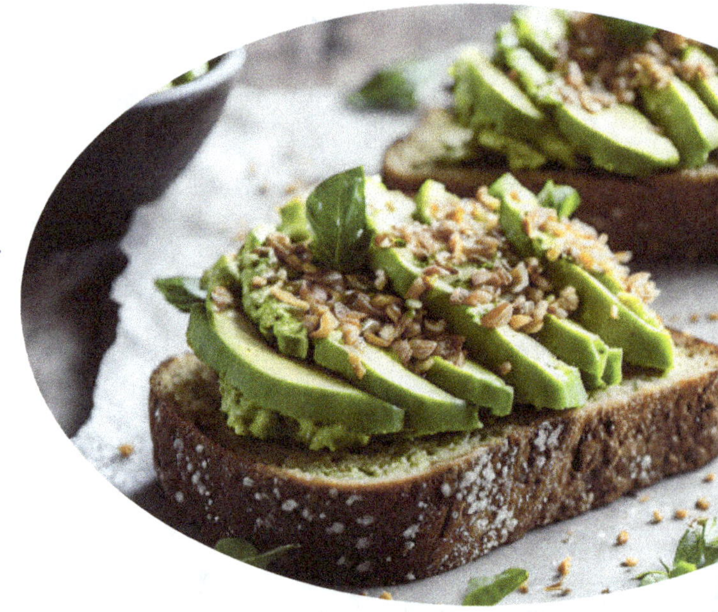

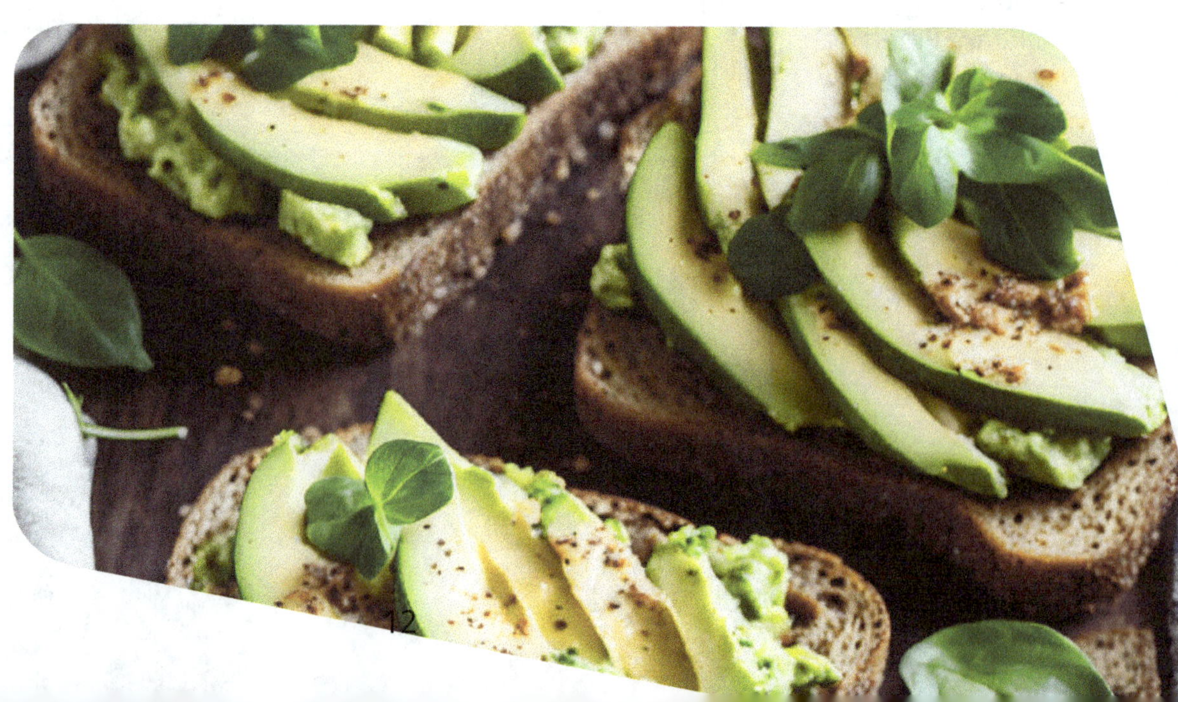

4. Spinach and Mushroom Omelette

Preparation Time: 10 minutes
Cook Time: 10 minutes
Total Time: 20 minutes

Serves: 1

Ingredients:

 3 large eggs
- 1 tablespoon unsalted butter
- 1/2 cup sliced mushrooms
- 1 cup fresh spinach leaves
- 2 tablespoons shredded cheddar cheese
- Salt and black pepper to taste

Directions:

1. Crack the eggs into a small bowl and beat them lightly with a fork until well combined.

2. Melt the butter in a small non-stick skillet over medium heat.

3. Add the sliced mushrooms to the skillet and cook for 2-3 minutes, stirring occasionally, until they start to soften.

4. Add the spinach leaves to the skillet and cook for 1-2 minutes, stirring frequently, until the spinach is wilted.

5. Pour the beaten eggs into the skillet and let them cook for 2-3 minutes, gently lifting the edges with a spatula to allow the uncooked egg to flow underneath.

6. When the eggs are mostly set but still a bit runny on top, sprinkle the shredded cheddar cheese over the top.

7. Fold the omelette in half and slide it onto a plate. Season with salt and black pepper to taste.

Nutrition Facts (per serving):
- Calories: 290
- Total Fat: 21g
- Saturated Fat: 9g
- Cholesterol: 435mg
- Sodium: 460mg
- Total Carbohydrates: 6g
- Dietary Fiber: 2g
- Sugars: 2g
- Protein: 21g

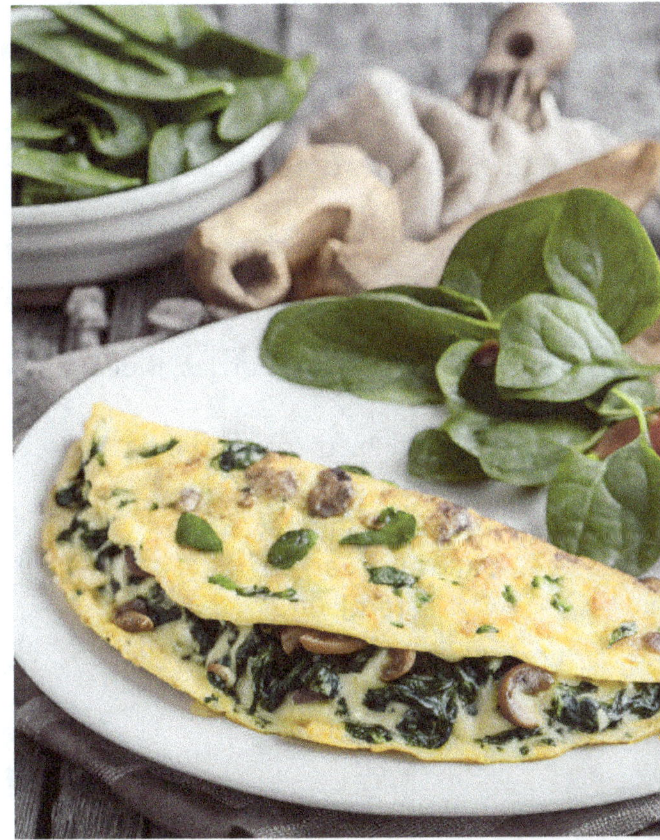

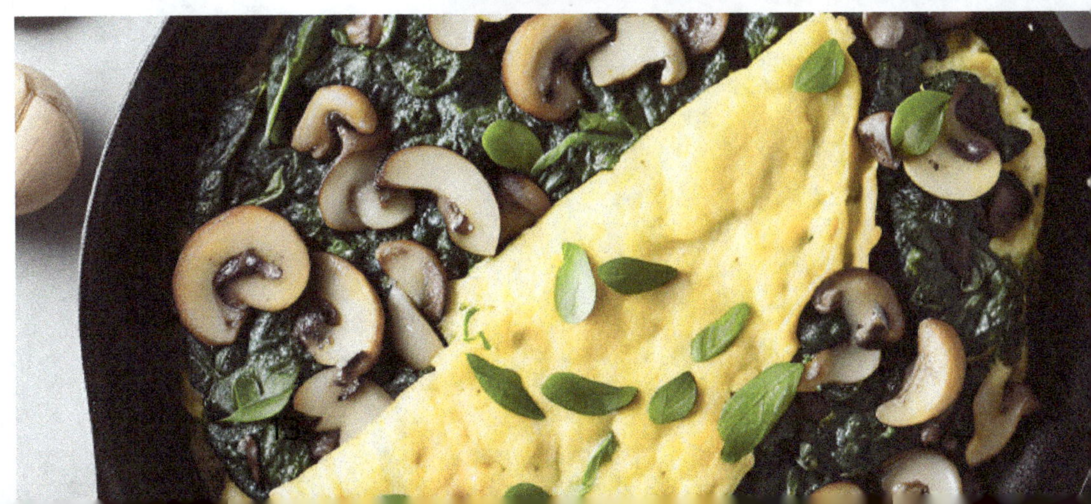

5. Chia Seed Pudding with Almond Milk

Preparation Time: 10 minutes
Chill Time: 4 hours or overnight
Total Time: 4 hours 10 minutes

Serves: 2

Directions:

1. In a medium bowl, whisk together the chia seeds, almond milk, maple syrup, and vanilla extract until well combined.

2. Cover the bowl and refrigerate for at least 4 hours or overnight, stirring occasionally, until the chia seeds have thickened the mixture into a pudding-like consistency.

3. Stir in the ground cinnamon, if using.

4. Divide the chia seed pudding between two serving bowls or jars.

5. Top with fresh berries, if desired.

Nutrition Facts (per serving):
- Calories: 150
- Total Fat: 8g
- Saturated Fat: 1g
- Cholesterol: 0mg
- Sodium: 75mg
- Total Carbohydrates: 18g
- Dietary Fiber: 9g
- Sugars: 8g
- Protein: 5g

Ingredients:

 1/4 cup chia seeds
- 1 cup unsweetened almond milk
- 1 tablespoon maple syrup (or honey)
- 1/2 teaspoon vanilla extract
- 1/4 teaspoon ground cinnamon (optional)
- Fresh berries, for serving (optional)

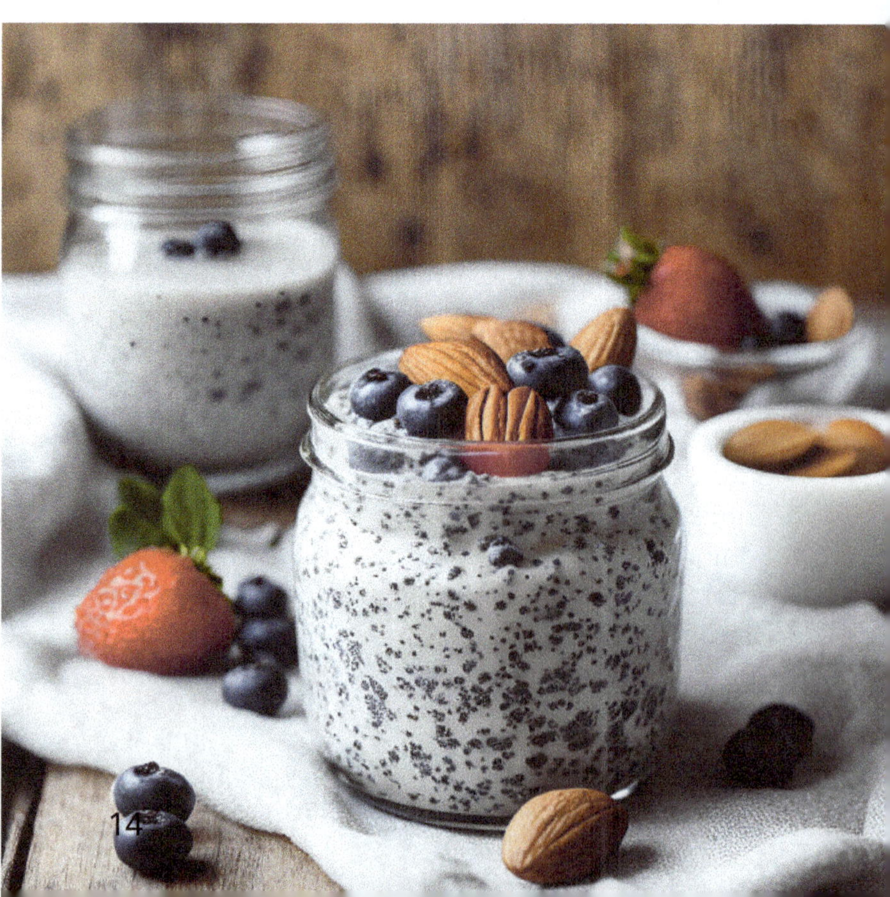

6. Smoothie Bowl with Spinach, Mango, and Protein Powder

Preparation Time: 10 minutes
Total Time: 10 minutes

Serves: 1

Directions:

1. In a high-speed blender, combine the spinach, frozen mango, almond milk, and protein powder. Blend until smooth and creamy.

2. Pour the smoothie into a serving bowl.

3. Top the smoothie with the chia seeds, sliced almonds, and shredded coconut.

Nutrition Facts (per serving):
- Calories: 350
- Total Fat: 15g
- Saturated Fat: 4g
- Cholesterol: 0mg
- Sodium: 160mg
- Total Carbohydrates: 37g
- Dietary Fiber: 10g
- Sugars: 20g
- Protein: 25g

Ingredients:

 1 cup fresh spinach leaves
- 1 cup frozen mango chunks
- 1/2 cup unsweetened almond milk
- 1 scoop vanilla protein powder
- 1 tablespoon chia seeds
- 1 tablespoon sliced almonds
- 1 tablespoon unsweetened shredded coconut

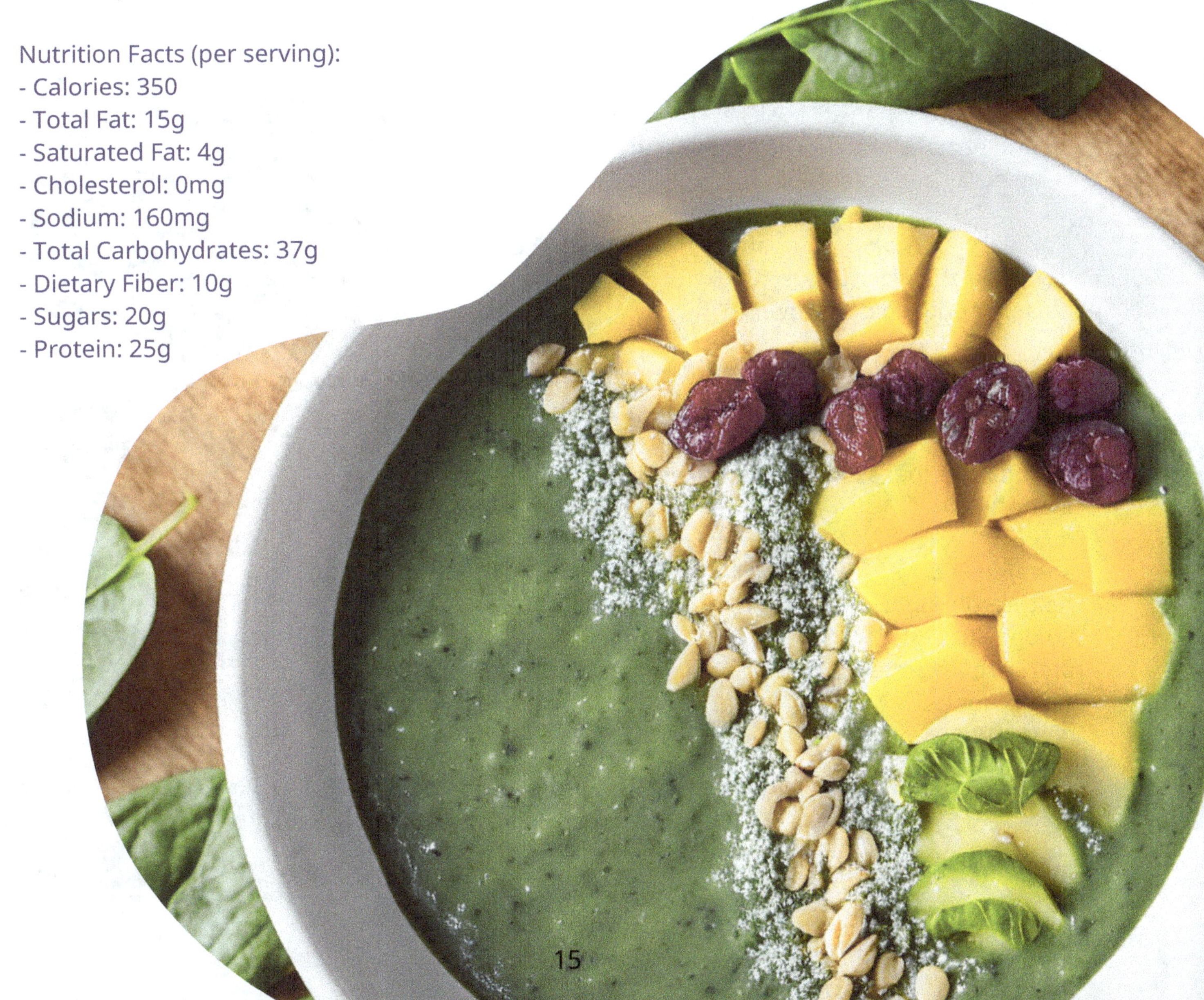

7. Whole Grain Pancakes with Blueberries

Preparation Time: 10 minutes
Cook Time: 15 minutes
Total Time: 25 minutes

Serves: 4 (makes 8 pancakes)

Directions:

1. In a medium bowl, whisk together the whole wheat flour, baking powder, baking soda, and salt.

2. In a separate bowl, whisk together the almond milk, egg, honey, and vanilla extract.

3. Pour the wet ingredients into the dry ingredients and stir just until combined (do not overmix).

4. Fold in the blueberries.

5. Heat a large non-stick skillet or griddle over medium heat. Lightly grease the surface with cooking spray or a small amount of oil.

6. For each pancake, pour about 1/4 cup of the batter onto the hot surface. Cook for 2-3 minutes per side, or until golden brown.

7. Serve the pancakes warm, with additional blueberries and maple syrup, if desired.

Nutrition Facts (per serving, 2 pancakes):
- Calories: 210
- Total Fat: 4g
- Saturated Fat: 1g
- Cholesterol: 55mg
- Sodium: 360mg
- Total Carbohydrates: 37g
- Dietary Fiber: 5g
- Sugars: 12g
- Protein: 8g

Ingredients:

 1 cup whole wheat flour
- 1 teaspoon baking powder
- 1/4 teaspoon baking soda
- 1/4 teaspoon salt
- 1 cup unsweetened almond milk
- 1 large egg
- 1 tablespoon honey
- 1 teaspoon vanilla extract
- 1 cup fresh or frozen blueberries

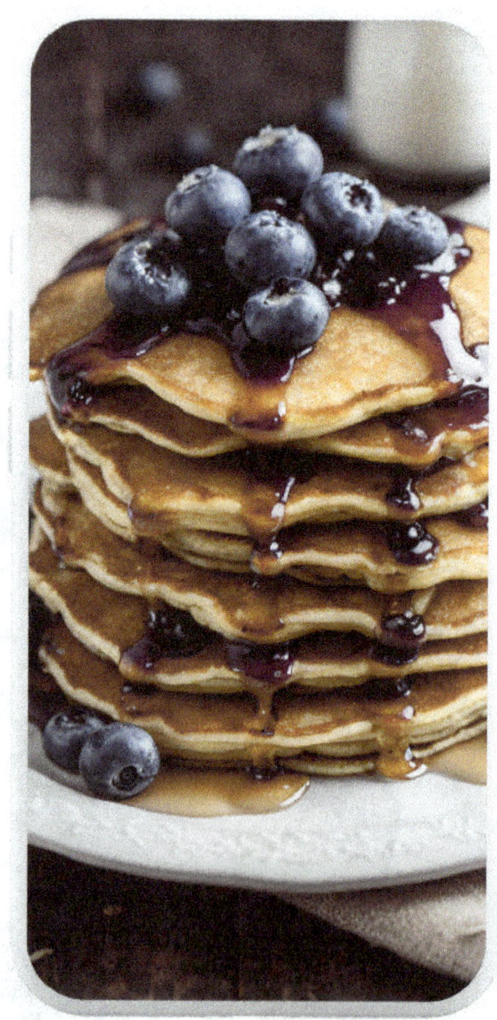

8. Quinoa Breakfast Bowl with Nuts and Fruits

Preparation Time: 10 minutes
Cook Time: 15 minutes
Total Time: 25 minutes

Serves: 1

Chapter 4 : Energizing Breakfast Recipes

Directions:

1. In a medium bowl, combine the cooked quinoa and almond milk. Stir to combine.

2. Top the quinoa mixture with the chopped walnuts, chopped almonds, and diced fresh fruit.

3. Drizzle the honey over the top, if using.

4. Sprinkle the ground cinnamon over the bowl.

5. Serve immediately.

Nutrition Facts (per serving):
- Calories: 320
- Total Fat: 16g
- Saturated Fat: 1.5g
- Cholesterol: 0mg
- Sodium: 45mg
- Total Carbohydrates: 38g
- Dietary Fiber: 7g
- Sugars: 12g
- Protein: 10g

Ingredients:

 1/2 cup cooked quinoa, cooled
- 1/2 cup unsweetened almond milk
- 1 tablespoon chopped walnuts
- 1 tablespoon chopped almonds
- 1/4 cup diced fresh fruit (such as strawberries, blueberries, or mango)
- 1 teaspoon honey (optional)
- Pinch of ground cinnamon

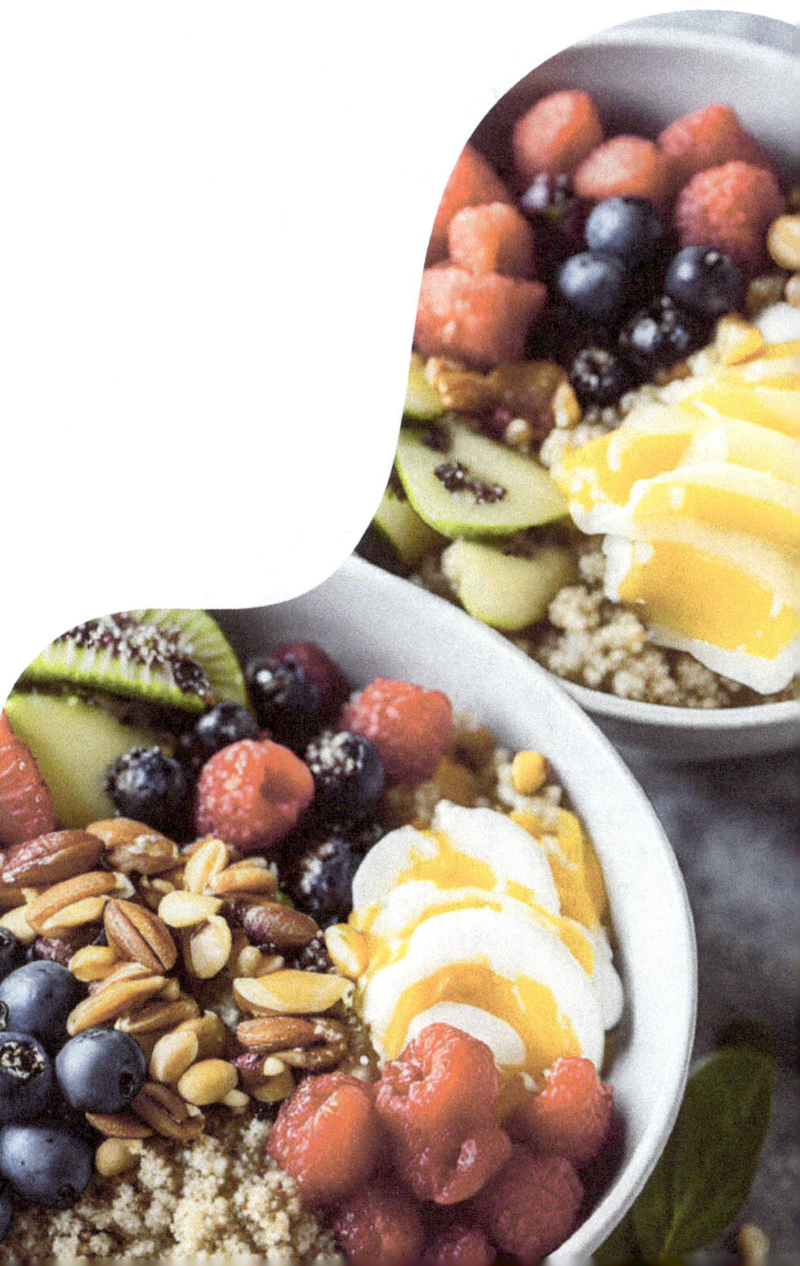

9. Sweet Potato and Black Bean Breakfast Burrito

Preparation Time: 15 minutes
Cook Time: 20 minutes
Total Time: 35 minutes

Serves: 4 burritos

Ingredients:

- 1 medium sweet potato, peeled and diced
- 1 tablespoon olive oil
- 1/2 teaspoon ground cumin
- 1/4 teaspoon chili powder
- Salt and pepper to taste
- 1 (15 oz) can black beans, drained and rinsed
- 4 large eggs, scrambled
- 4 whole wheat tortillas
- 1/4 cup shredded cheddar cheese

Directions:

1. Preheat the oven to 400°F. Toss the diced sweet potato with the olive oil, cumin, chili powder, salt, and pepper. Spread the sweet potato on a baking sheet and roast for 15-20 minutes, until tender.

2. In a medium skillet, heat the black beans over medium heat until warmed through.

3. In a separate skillet, scramble the eggs until cooked through.

4. To assemble the burritos, place a tortilla on a flat surface. Layer the roasted sweet potato, black beans, and scrambled eggs down the center. Top with shredded cheddar cheese.

5. Fold the bottom of the tortilla up over the filling, then fold in the sides and continue rolling up tightly into a burrito.

6. Repeat with the remaining ingredients to make 4 burritos.

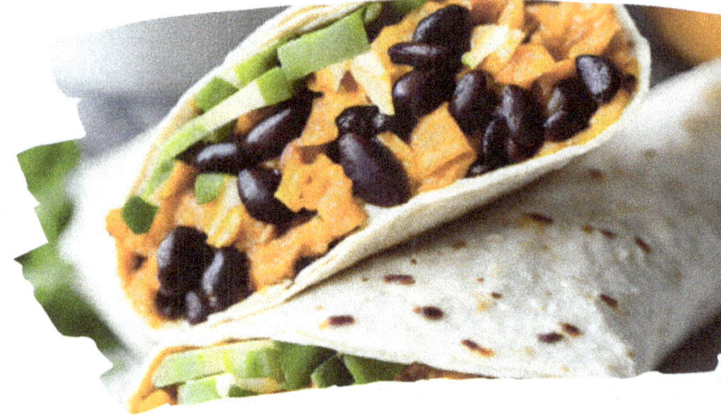

Nutrition Facts (per burrito):
- Calories: 350
- Total Fat: 13g
- Saturated Fat: 4g
- Cholesterol: 190mg
- Sodium: 590mg
- Total Carbohydrates: 44g
- Dietary Fiber: 8g
- Sugars: 3g
- Protein: 16g

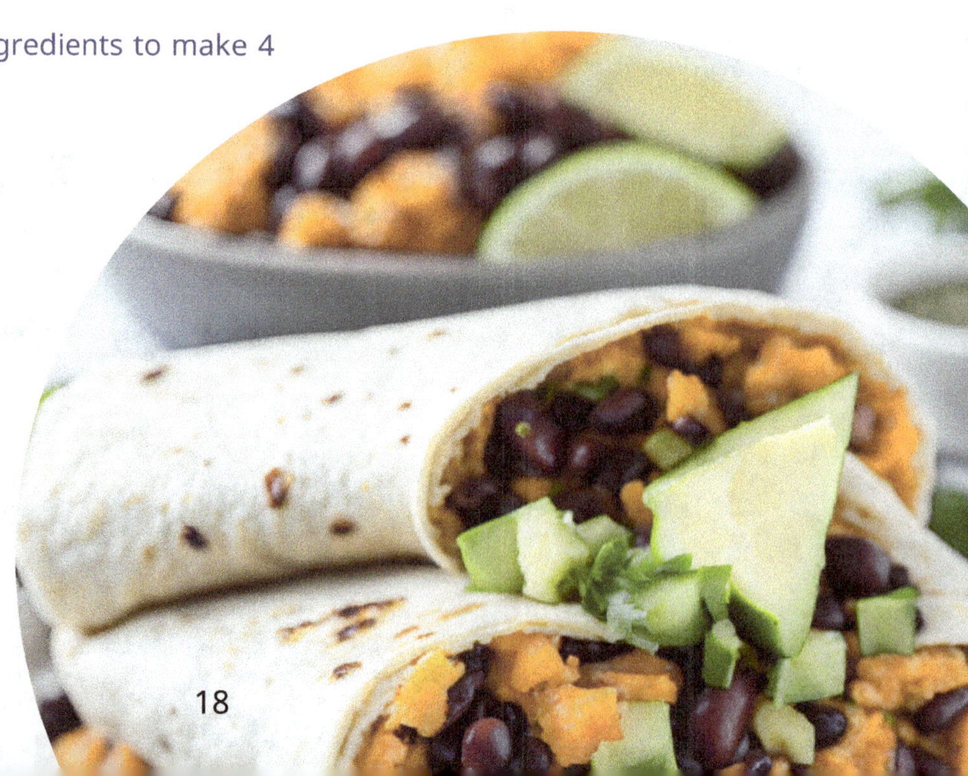

10. Almond Butter and Banana on Rye Bread

Preparation Time: 5 minutes
Cook Time: 0 minutes
Total Time: 5 minutes

Serves: 1

Ingredients:

 2 slices rye bread
- 2 tablespoons creamy almond butter
- 1 ripe banana, sliced

Directions:

1. Toast the rye bread slices until lightly golden.

2. Spread the almond butter evenly over one side of each toast slice.

3. Arrange the sliced banana over the almond butter.

4. Serve immediately.

Nutrition Facts (per serving, 2 slices):
- Calories: 350
- Total Fat: 18g
- Saturated Fat: 2g
- Cholesterol: 0mg
- Sodium: 360mg
- Total Carbohydrates: 43g
- Dietary Fiber: 7g
- Sugars: 13g
- Protein: 10g

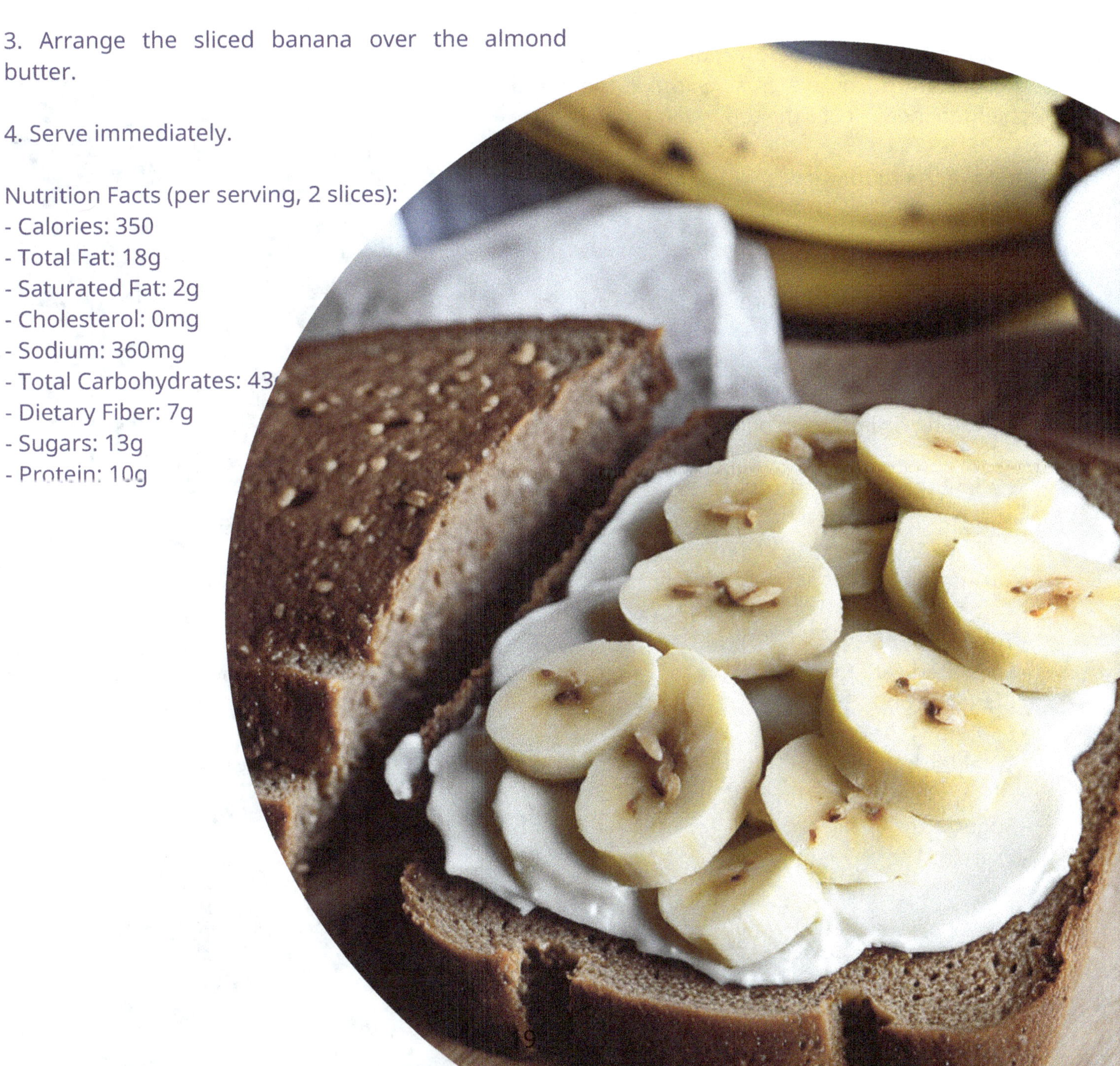

11. Breakfast Quiche with Broccoli and Cheese

Preparation Time: 20 minutes
Cook Time: 40 minutes
Total Time: 1 hour

Serves: 6

Directions:

1. Preheat the oven to 375°F.

2. Press the pie crust into a 9-inch pie plate and crimp the edges.

3. Spread the chopped broccoli florets evenly over the bottom of the pie crust. Sprinkle the shredded cheddar cheese over the top.

4. In a medium bowl, whisk together the eggs, almond milk, salt, and black pepper until well combined.

5. Pour the egg mixture over the broccoli and cheese in the pie crust.

6. Bake for 40-45 minutes, or until the center is set and the top is lightly golden.

7. Allow the quiche to cool for 5-10 minutes before slicing and serving.

Nutrition Facts (per serving):
- Calories: 280
- Total Fat: 18g
- Saturated Fat: 7g
- Cholesterol: 215mg
- Sodium: 430mg
- Total Carbohydrates: 18g
- Dietary Fiber: 2g
- Sugars: 2g
- Protein: 13g

Ingredients:

 1 pre-made 9-inch pie crust
- 1 cup chopped broccoli florets
- 1/2 cup shredded cheddar cheese
- 6 large eggs
- 1 cup unsweetened almond milk
- 1/4 teaspoon salt
- 1/4 teaspoon black pepper

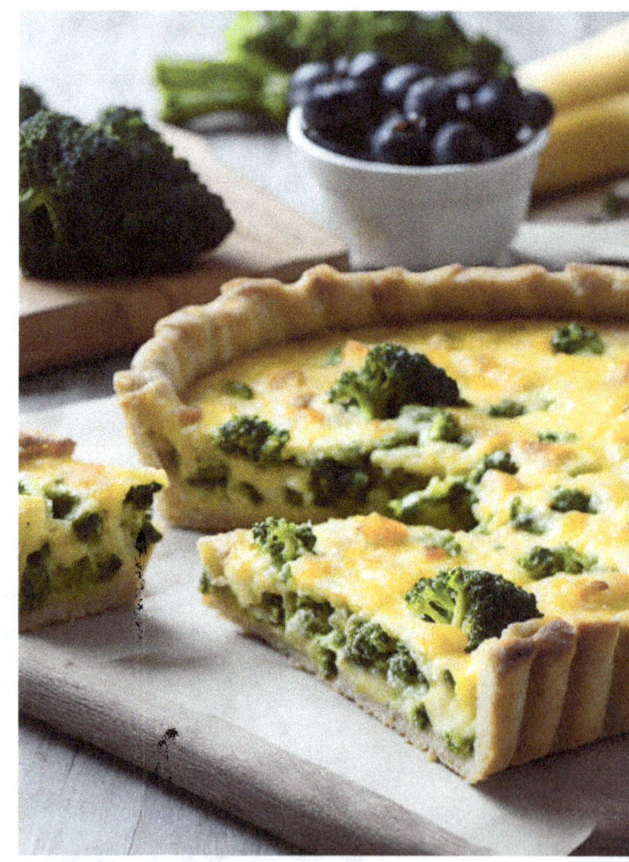

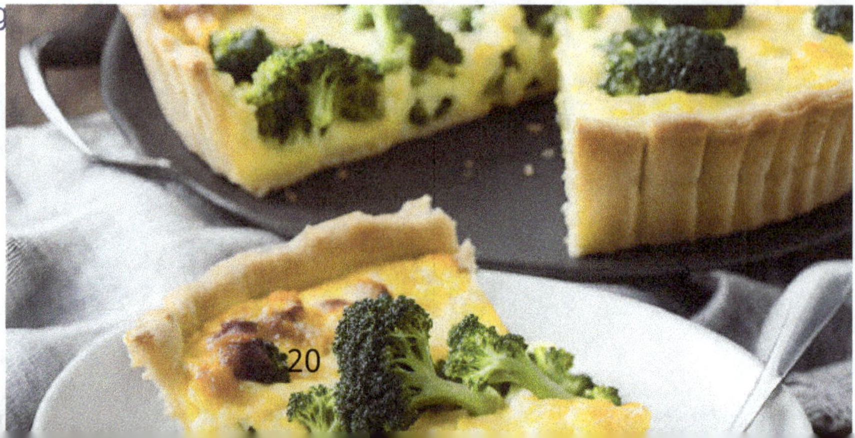

12. Egg Muffins with Veggies

Preparation Time: 15 minutes
Cook Time: 25 minutes
Total Time: 40 minutes

Serves: 6 (makes 12 muffins)

Ingredients:

8 large eggs
- 1/2 cup unsweetened almond milk
- 1/4 teaspoon salt
- 1/4 teaspoon black pepper
- 1 cup diced bell peppers
- 1/2 cup diced onions
- 1 cup chopped spinach
- 1/2 cup shredded cheddar cheese

Directions:

1. Preheat the oven to 375°F. Grease a 12-cup muffin tin with non-stick cooking spray.

2. In a large bowl, whisk together the eggs, almond milk, salt, and black pepper until well combined.

3. Stir in the diced bell peppers, diced onions, and chopped spinach.

4. Divide the egg mixture evenly among the 12 muffin cups. Sprinkle the shredded cheddar cheese over the top.

5. Bake for 22-25 minutes, or until the eggs are set and the tops are lightly golden.

6. Allow the egg muffins to cool in the tin for 5 minutes before removing them.

7. Serve warm or at room temperature.

Nutrition Facts (per muffin):
- Calories: 100
- Total Fat: 6g
- Saturated Fat: 3g
- Cholesterol: 160mg
- Sodium: 240mg
- Total Carbohydrates: 3g
- Dietary Fiber: 1g
- Sugars: 1g
- Protein: 8g

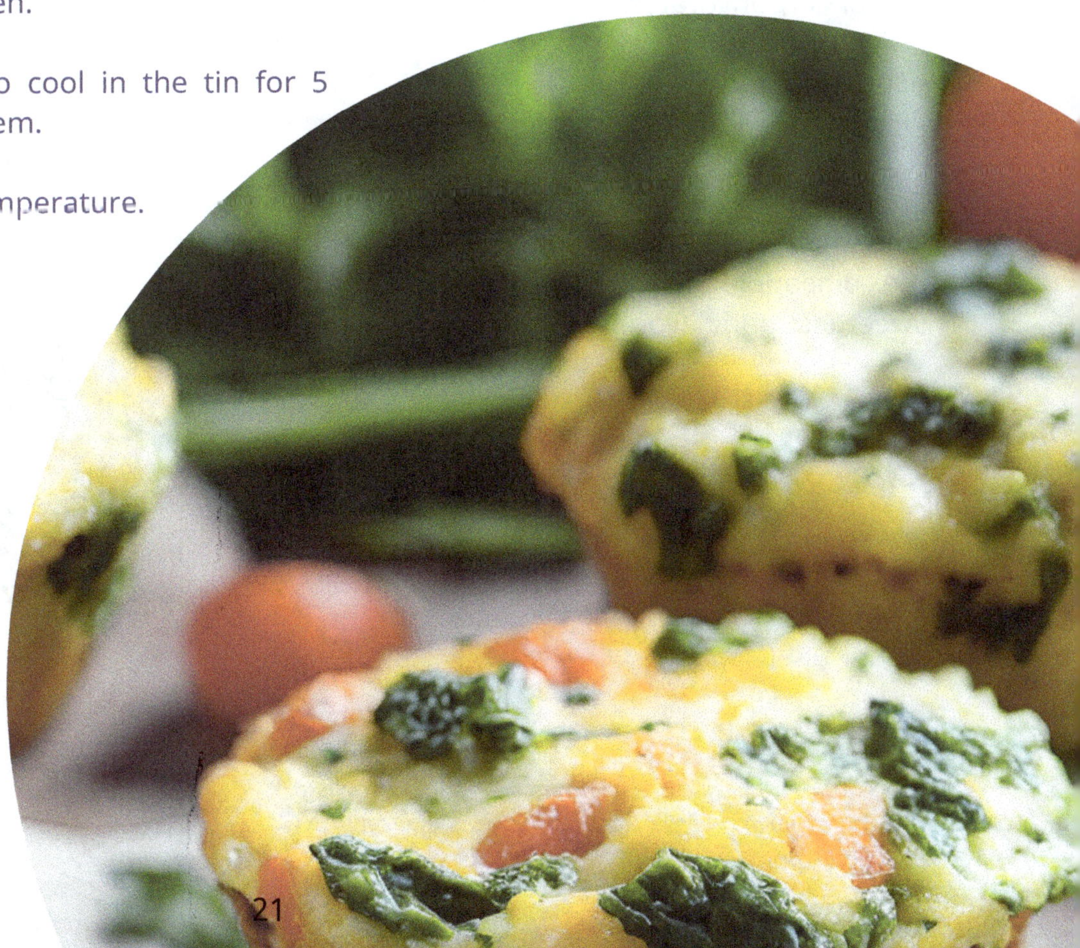

13. Turmeric Smoothie with Pineapple

Preparation Time: 5 minutes
Total Time: 5 minutes

Serves: 1

Directions:

1. Add all the ingredients to a high-speed blender.

2. Blend on high speed until smooth and creamy, about 1 minute.

3. Pour the smoothie into a glass and enjoy immediately.

Nutrition Facts (per serving):
- Calories: 200
- Total Fat: 2g
- Saturated Fat: 0g
- Cholesterol: 0mg
- Sodium: 65mg
- Total Carbohydrates: 46g
- Dietary Fiber: 4g
- Sugars: 36g
- Protein: 3g

The turmeric, ginger, and black pepper in this smoothie provide anti-inflammatory benefits, while the pineapple and honey (if used) add natural sweetness and flavor.

Ingredients:
 1 cup frozen pineapple chunks
- 1 cup unsweetened almond milk
- 1 tablespoon ground turmeric
- 1 tablespoon honey (optional)
- 1/2 teaspoon ground ginger
- 1/4 teaspoon ground black pepper

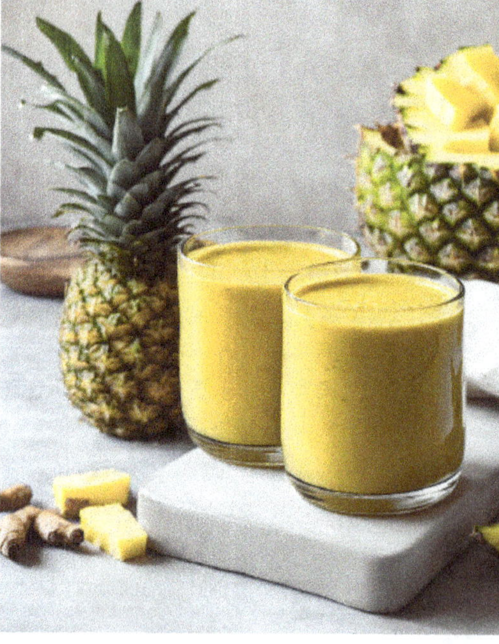

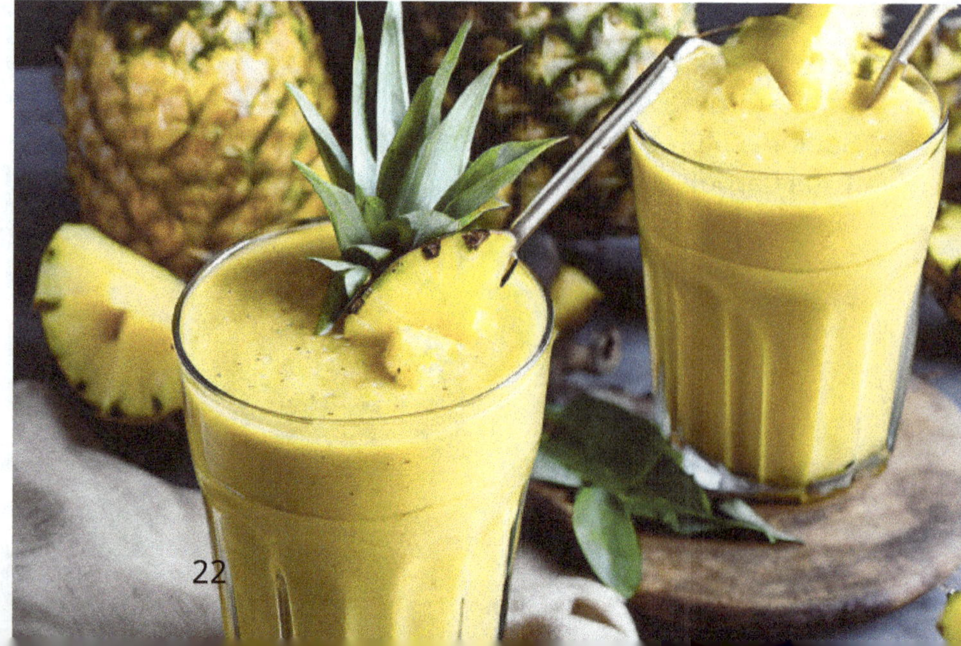

14. Apple Cinnamon Overnight Oats

Preparation Time: 10 minutes
Chill Time: 8 hours or overnight
Total Time: 8 hours 10 minutes

Serves: 1

Ingredients:

1/2 cup old-fashioned rolled oats
- 1/2 cup unsweetened almond milk
- 2 tablespoons plain Greek yogurt
- 1 tablespoon chia seeds
- 1 teaspoon maple syrup
- 1/2 teaspoon ground cinnamon
- 1/4 teaspoon vanilla extract
- 1/2 cup diced apple

Directions:

1. In a mason jar or airtight container, combine the rolled oats, almond milk, Greek yogurt, chia seeds, maple syrup, cinnamon, and vanilla extract. Stir until well mixed.

2. Fold in the diced apple.

3. Cover and refrigerate for at least 8 hours or overnight.

4. When ready to serve, give the overnight oats a stir and enjoy chilled.

Nutrition Facts (per serving):
- Calories: 300
- Total Fat: 9g
- Saturated Fat: 1.5g
- Cholesterol: 5mg
- Sodium: 65mg
- Total Carbohydrates: 45g
- Dietary Fiber: 8g
- Sugars: 15g
- Protein: 12g

The combination of oats, Greek yogurt, chia seeds, and apples provides a nutritious and filling breakfast that's easy to prepare ahead of time.

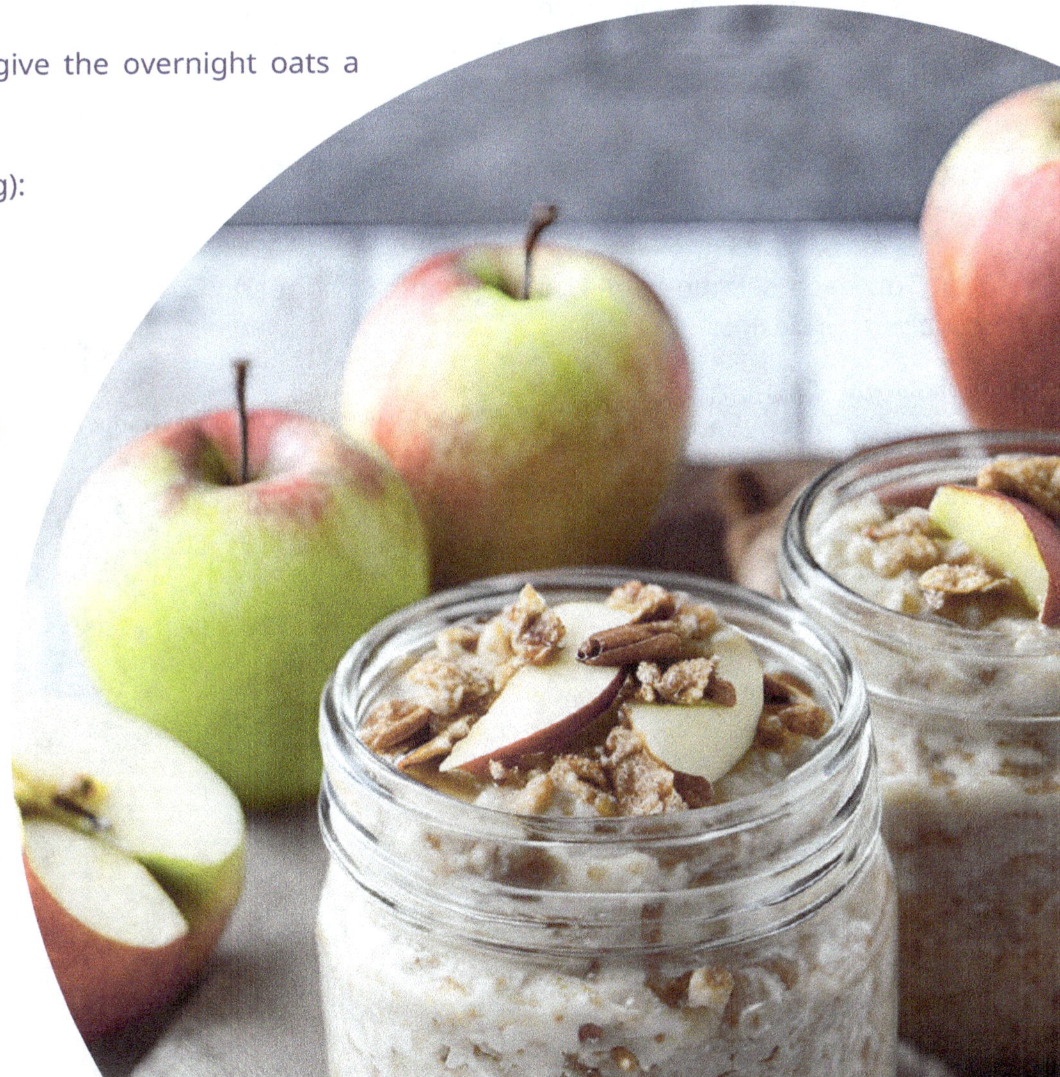

15. Buckwheat Porridge with Maple Syrup

Preparation Time: 5 minutes
Cook Time: 15 minutes
Total Time: 20 minutes

Serves: 2

Directions:

1. In a small saucepan, combine the almond milk and buckwheat groats. Bring the mixture to a simmer over medium heat.

2. Reduce the heat to low and let the buckwheat simmer, stirring occasionally, for 12-15 minutes, until the groats are tender and the porridge has thickened.

3. Remove the saucepan from the heat and stir in the maple syrup, cinnamon, vanilla extract, and a pinch of salt.

4. Divide the buckwheat porridge between two serving bowls.

5. Top each serving with 1 tablespoon of chopped walnuts, if desired.

6. Serve warm.

Nutrition Facts (per serving):
- Calories: 200
- Total Fat: 7g
- Saturated Fat: 1g
- Cholesterol: 0mg
- Sodium: 75mg
- Total Carbohydrates: 29g
- Dietary Fiber: 4g
- Sugars: 10g
- Protein: 5g

Buckwheat is a gluten-free grain that provides fiber, protein, and essential nutrients. The maple syrup and cinnamon add natural sweetness and flavor to this nourishing breakfast porridge.

Ingredients:

1 cup unsweetened almond milk
- 1/2 cup raw buckwheat groats
- 1 tablespoon maple syrup
- 1/4 teaspoon ground cinnamon
- 1/4 teaspoon vanilla extract
- Pinch of salt
- 2 tablespoons chopped walnuts (optional)

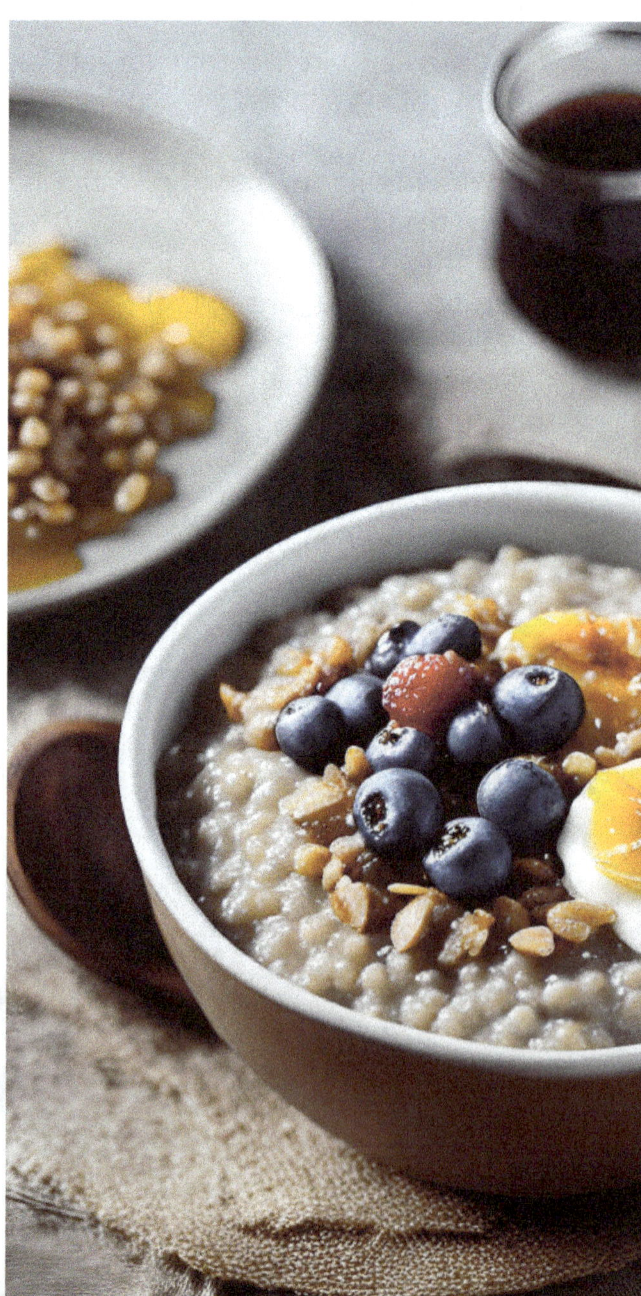

16. Greek Yogurt Parfait with Granola and Cherries

Preparation Time: 10 minutes
Total Time: 10 minutes

Serves: 1

Ingredients:

 1 cup plain Greek yogurt
- 1/2 cup fresh or frozen pitted cherries
- 1/4 cup granola
- 1 teaspoon honey (optional)

Directions:

1. In a parfait glass or bowl, layer half of the Greek yogurt.

2. Top the yogurt with half of the cherries.

3. Sprinkle half of the granola over the cherries.

4. Repeat the layers, ending with the remaining granola.

5. Drizzle the honey over the top, if using.

6. Serve immediately.

Nutrition Facts (per serving):
- Calories: 300
- Total Fat: 8g
- Saturated Fat: 2g
- Cholesterol: 25mg
- Sodium: 105mg
- Total Carbohydrates: 37g
- Dietary Fiber: 5g
- Sugars: 24g
- Protein: 20g

The combination of protein-rich Greek yogurt, fiber-filled granola, and antioxidant-packed cherries makes this a nutritious and satisfying breakfast or snack. The honey adds a touch of sweetness if desired.

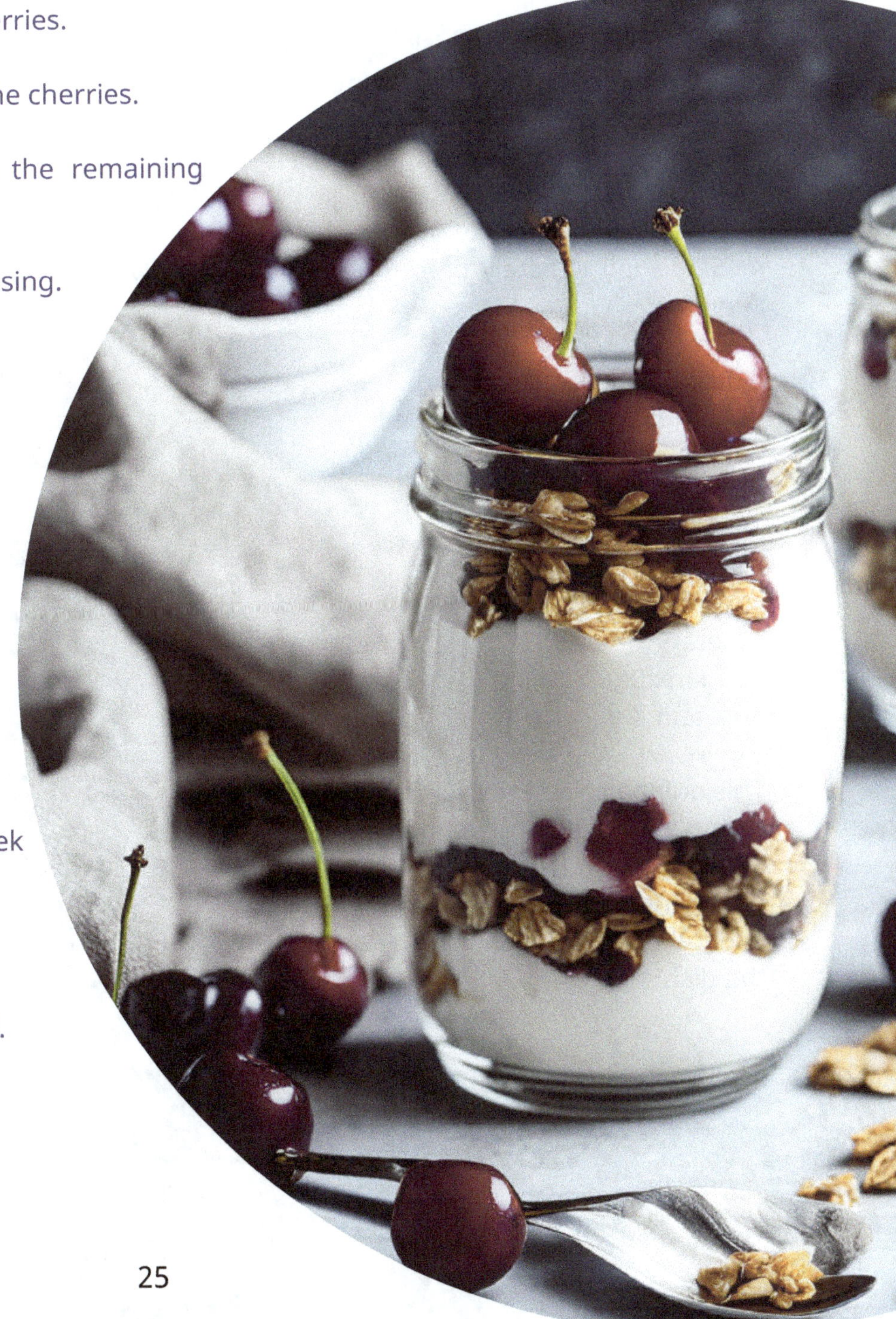

1. Quinoa Salad with Chickpeas and Avocado

Preparation Time: 15 minutes
Total Time: 15 minutes

Serves: 4

Directions:

1. In a large bowl, combine the cooked quinoa, chickpeas, diced avocado, cucumber, red onion, and chopped cilantro.

2. In a small bowl, whisk together the olive oil, lemon juice, salt, and black pepper.

3. Pour the dressing over the quinoa salad and toss gently to coat.

4. Serve immediately or refrigerate until ready to serve.

Ingredients:

1 cup cooked quinoa, cooled
- 1 (15 oz) can chickpeas, drained and rinsed
- 1 avocado, diced
- 1/2 cup diced cucumber
- 1/4 cup diced red onion
- 2 tablespoons chopped fresh cilantro
- 2 tablespoons olive oil
- 2 tablespoons lemon juice
- 1/4 teaspoon salt
- 1/4 teaspoon black pepper

Nutrition Facts (per serving):
- Calories: 300
- Total Fat: 15g
- Saturated Fat: 2g
- Cholesterol: 0mg
- Sodium: 360mg
- Total Carbohydrates: 35g
- Dietary Fiber: 9g
- Sugars: 3g
- Protein: 9g

This quinoa salad is packed with plant-based protein, healthy fats, and fiber. The avocado and lemon juice dressing add creaminess and freshness to the dish.

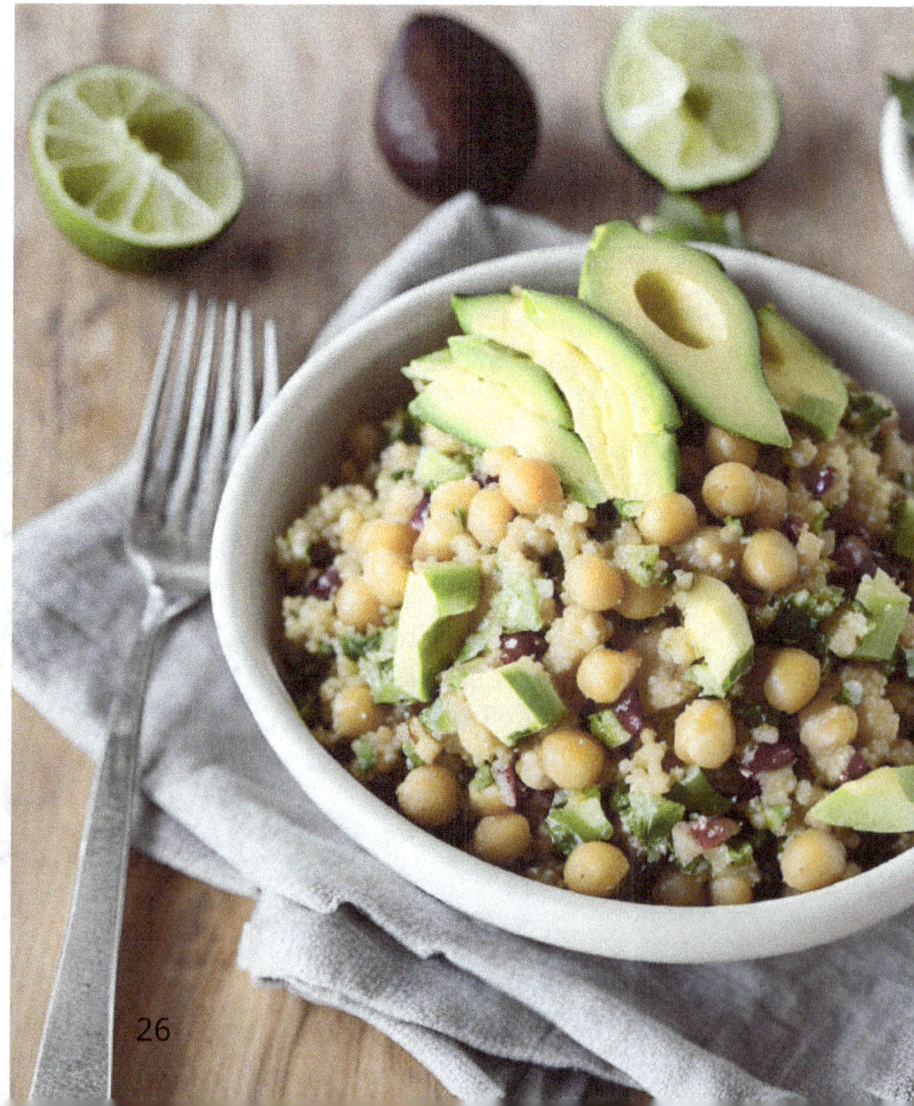

2. Grilled Chicken and Vegetable Wrap

Preparation Time: 15 minutes
Cook Time: 10 minutes
Total Time: 25 minutes

Serves: 4 wraps

Ingredients:

4 whole wheat tortillas or wraps
- 1 lb boneless, skinless chicken breasts
- 1 tablespoon olive oil
- 1 teaspoon dried Italian seasoning
- Salt and pepper to taste
- 1 cup sliced bell peppers
- 1/2 cup sliced cucumber
- 1/2 cup shredded carrots
- 2 tablespoons hummus
- 2 tablespoons crumbled feta cheese (optional)

Directions:

1. Preheat grill or grill pan to medium-high heat.
2. Brush the chicken breasts with olive oil and season with the Italian seasoning, salt, and pepper.
3. Grill the chicken for 5-7 minutes per side, or until cooked through. Let rest for 5 minutes, then slice or shred the chicken.
4. Warm the tortillas according to package instructions.
5. Spread 1/2 tablespoon of hummus down the center of each tortilla.
6. Top with the grilled chicken, sliced bell peppers, cucumber, and shredded carrots.
7. Sprinkle the feta cheese over the top, if using.
8. Fold the bottom of the tortilla up over the filling, then fold in the sides and continue rolling up tightly into a wrap.

Nutrition Facts (per wrap):
- Calories: 350
- Total Fat: 12g
- Saturated Fat: 2.5g
- Cholesterol: 65mg
- Sodium: 550mg
- Total Carbohydrates: 35g
- Dietary Fiber: 6g
- Sugars: 4g
- Protein: 28g

This wrap is a great balance of lean protein, vegetables, and whole grains. The hummus and feta add extra flavor and creaminess.

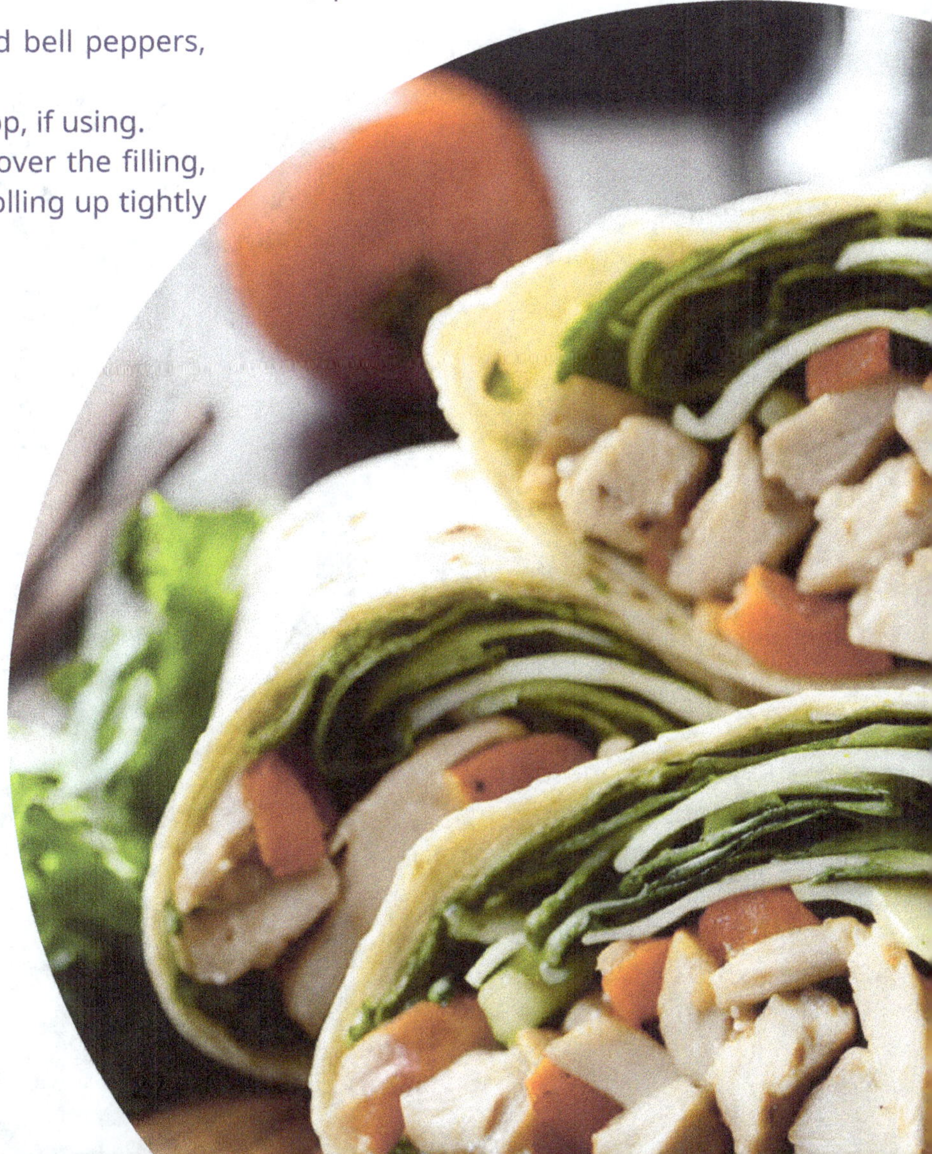

3. Lentil Soup with Spinach and Carrots

Preparation Time: 15 minutes
Cook Time: 30 minutes
Total Time: 45 minutes

Serves: 4

Directions:

1. In a large pot or Dutch oven, heat the olive oil over medium heat. Add the diced onion and carrots and cook for 5-7 minutes, until softened.
2. Add the minced garlic and cook for 1 minute, until fragrant.
3. Stir in the rinsed lentils, vegetable broth, diced tomatoes, cumin, thyme, and red pepper flakes (if using). Season with salt and black pepper.
4. Bring the soup to a boil, then reduce the heat and let it simmer for 20-25 minutes, or until the lentils are tender.
5. Stir in the fresh spinach leaves and cook for 2-3 minutes more, until the spinach is wilted.
6. Taste and adjust seasoning as needed.
7. Serve the lentil soup hot.

Nutrition Facts (per serving):
- Calories: 280
- Total Fat: 6g
- Saturated Fat: 1g
- Cholesterol: 0mg
- Sodium: 480mg
- Total Carbohydrates: 42g
- Dietary Fiber: 13g
- Sugars: 8g
- Protein: 16g

This hearty lentil soup is a nutritious and filling vegetarian meal. The spinach and carrots add extra vitamins and fiber.

Ingredients:

 1 tablespoon olive oil
- 1 onion, diced
- 3 carrots, peeled and diced
- 3 cloves garlic, minced
- 1 cup dried brown lentils, rinsed
- 4 cups low-sodium vegetable broth
- 1 (14.5 oz) can diced tomatoes
- 1 teaspoon ground cumin
- 1/2 teaspoon dried thyme
- 1/4 teaspoon red pepper flakes (optional)
- Salt and black pepper to taste
- 2 cups fresh spinach leaves

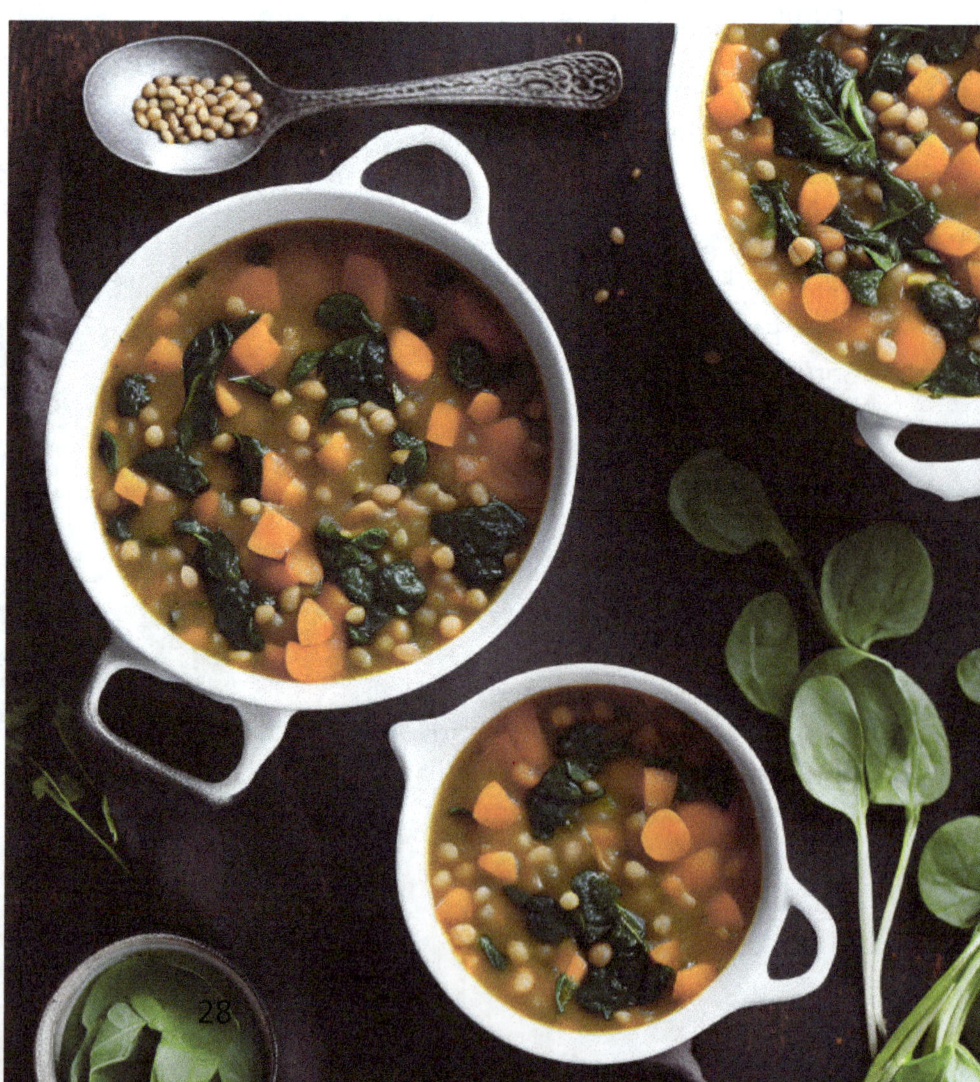

4. Kale and Sweet Potato Salad with Lemon Dressing

Preparation Time: 20 minutes
Cook Time: 20 minutes
Total Time: 40 minutes

Serves: 4

Ingredients:

For the Salad:
- 1 medium sweet potato, peeled and diced
- 1 tablespoon olive oil
- 4 cups chopped kale, stems removed
- 1 (15 oz) can chickpeas, drained and rinsed
- 1/4 cup toasted pumpkin seeds

For the Dressing:
- 2 tablespoons lemon juice
- 1 tablespoon olive oil
- 1 teaspoon Dijon mustard
- 1 teaspoon honey
- 1/4 teaspoon salt
- 1/4 teaspoon black pepper

Directions:

1. Preheat the oven to 400°F. Toss the diced sweet potato with 1 tablespoon of olive oil and spread on a baking sheet. Roast for 18-20 minutes, until tender.

2. In a large bowl, combine the roasted sweet potato, chopped kale, chickpeas, and toasted pumpkin seeds.

3. In a small bowl, whisk together the lemon juice, 1 tablespoon olive oil, Dijon mustard, honey, salt, and black pepper to make the dressing.

4. Pour the dressing over the salad and toss to coat.

5. Serve immediately or refrigerate until ready to serve.

Nutrition Facts (per serving):
- Calories: 260
- Total Fat: 12g
- Saturated Fat: 2g
- Cholesterol: 0mg
- Sodium: 360mg
- Total Carbohydrates: 32g
- Dietary Fiber: 8g
- Sugars: 7g
- Protein: 9g

This salad is packed with nutrient-dense ingredients like kale, sweet potato, and chickpeas. The lemon dressing adds a bright, tangy flavor.

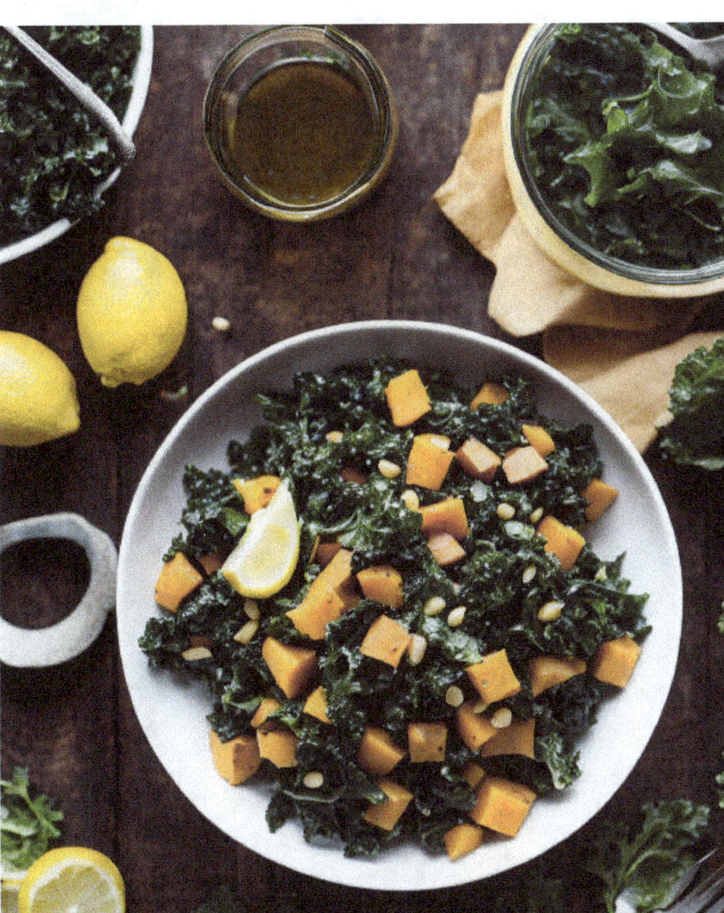

5. Turkey and Avocado Sandwich on Whole Grain Bread

Preparation Time: 5 minutes
Total Time: 5 minutes

Serves: 1

Ingredients:

 2 slices whole grain bread
- 2-3 ounces sliced turkey breast
- 1/2 avocado, sliced
- 1 tomato slice
- 1 leaf of lettuce
- 1 tablespoon hummus
- Salt and pepper to taste

Directions:

1. Spread the hummus evenly on one slice of the whole grain bread.

2. Layer the sliced turkey, avocado, tomato, and lettuce on top of the hummus.

3. Season with salt and pepper.

4. Top with the other slice of whole grain bread.

5. Cut the sandwich in half and serve.

Nutrition Facts (per sandwich):
- Calories: 350
- Total Fat: 16g
- Saturated Fat: 2.5g
- Cholesterol: 30mg
- Sodium: 650mg
- Total Carbohydrates: 35g
- Dietary Fiber: 9g
- Sugars: 4g
- Protein: 22g

This sandwich provides a balance of lean protein, healthy fats, and complex carbohydrates. The whole grain bread, avocado, and hummus make it a nutritious and satisfying lunch option.

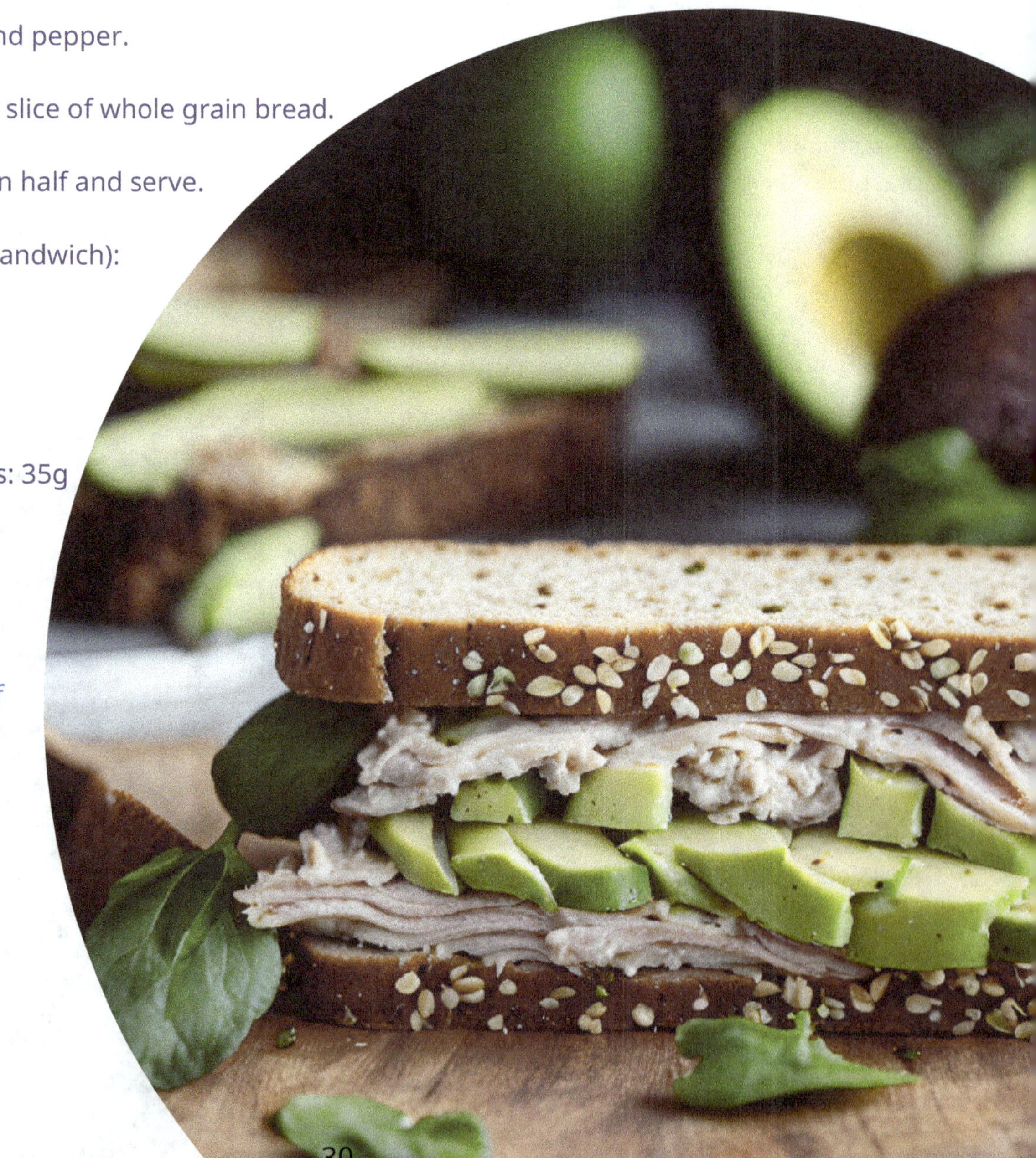

6. Tofu and Veggie Stir-fry

Preparation Time: 15 minutes
Cook Time: 15 minutes
Total Time: 30 minutes

Serves: 4

Directions:

1. In a large skillet or wok, heat 1 tablespoon of the sesame oil over medium-high heat. Add the cubed tofu and cook, stirring occasionally, until lightly browned on all sides, about 5-7 minutes. Transfer the tofu to a plate.
2. In the same skillet, heat the remaining 1 tablespoon of sesame oil. Add the broccoli, bell pepper, and mushrooms. Stir-fry for 5-7 minutes, until the vegetables are tender-crisp.
3. Add the garlic and ginger to the skillet and cook for 1 minute, until fragrant.
4. In a small bowl, whisk together the soy sauce, rice vinegar, honey, and red pepper flakes (if using).
5. Add the cooked tofu back to the skillet and pour the soy sauce mixture over the top. Toss everything together and cook for 2-3 minutes, until the sauce has thickened slightly.
6. Serve the tofu and veggie stir-fry over the cooked brown rice.

Nutrition Facts (per serving, 1/4 of recipe):
- Calories: 320
- Total Fat: 15g
- Saturated Fat: 2g
- Cholesterol: 0mg
- Sodium: 480mg
- Total Carbohydrates: 32g
- Dietary Fiber: 5g
- Sugars: 6g
- Protein: 18g

This stir-fry is a great way to incorporate plant-based protein from tofu and plenty of nutrient-dense vegetables. Serve it over whole grain brown rice for a complete and satisfying meal.

Ingredients:

 1 block (14 oz) extra-firm tofu, cubed
- 2 tablespoons sesame oil, divided
- 2 cups broccoli florets
- 1 red bell pepper, sliced
- 1 cup sliced mushrooms
- 2 cloves garlic, minced
- 1 tablespoon grated fresh ginger
- 2 tablespoons low-sodium soy sauce
- 1 tablespoon rice vinegar
- 1 teaspoon honey
- 1/4 teaspoon red pepper flakes (optional)
- 2 cups cooked brown rice, for serving

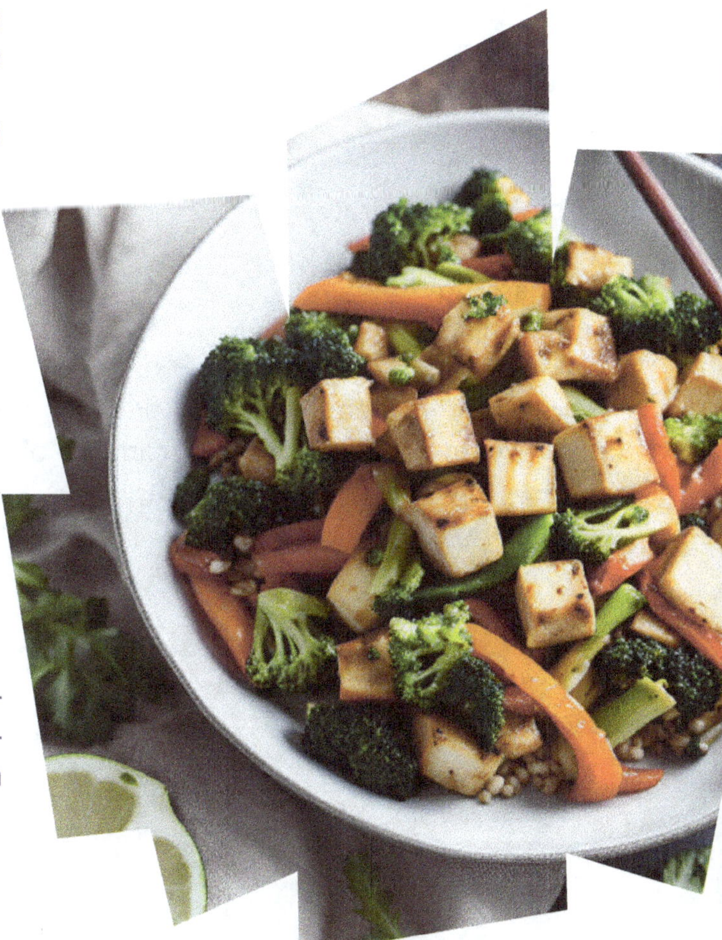

7. Mediterranean Salad with Feta and Olives

Preparation Time: 15 minutes
Total Time: 15 minutes

Serves: 4

Directions:

1. In a large salad bowl, combine the mixed greens, cherry tomatoes, diced cucumber, kalamata olives, crumbled feta, and chopped parsley.

2. In a small bowl, whisk together the olive oil, red wine vinegar, Dijon mustard, minced garlic, and dried oregano. Season with salt and pepper.

3. Drizzle the dressing over the salad and toss gently to coat.

4. Serve immediately.

Nutrition Facts (per serving):
- Calories: 180
- Total Fat: 14g
- Saturated Fat: 4g
- Cholesterol: 15mg
- Sodium: 420mg
- Total Carbohydrates: 10g
- Dietary Fiber: 3g
- Sugars: 4g
- Protein: 6g

This Mediterranean-inspired salad is packed with fresh vegetables, healthy fats from the olive oil and olives, and tangy feta cheese. It makes a light and refreshing lunch or side dish.

Ingredients:

5 cups mixed greens (such as spinach, arugula, and romaine)
- 1 cup cherry tomatoes, halved
- 1/2 cup diced cucumber
- 1/4 cup pitted kalamata olives, halved
- 1/4 cup crumbled feta cheese
- 2 tablespoons chopped fresh parsley
- 2 tablespoons olive oil
- 1 tablespoon red wine vinegar
- 1 teaspoon Dijon mustard
- 1 clove garlic, minced
- 1/4 teaspoon dried oregano
- Salt and pepper to taste

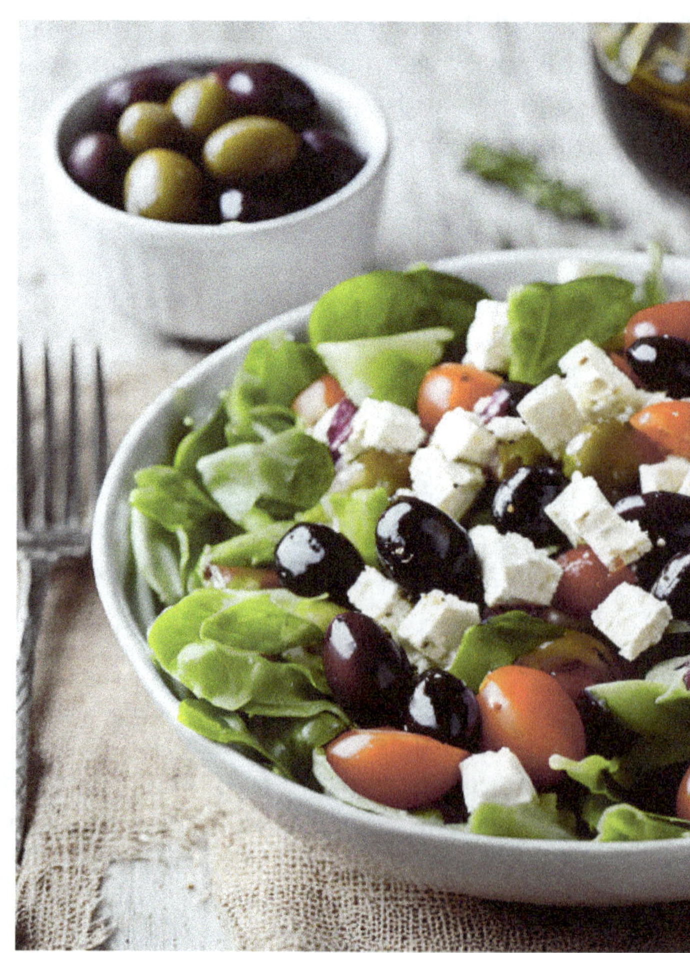

8. Butternut Squash Soup

Preparation Time: 20 minutes
Cook Time: 45 minutes
Total Time: 1 hour 5 minutes

Serves: 4

Directions:

1. Preheat the oven to 400°F. Toss the cubed butternut squash with the olive oil and spread on a baking sheet. Roast for 25-30 minutes, until tender.
2. In a large pot or Dutch oven, sauté the diced onion in a bit of olive oil over medium heat for 5-7 minutes, until translucent.
3. Add the minced garlic and cook for 1 minute, until fragrant.
4. Add the roasted butternut squash, vegetable broth, cumin, cinnamon, and nutmeg. Season with salt and black pepper.
5. Bring the soup to a boil, then reduce the heat and let it simmer for 15-20 minutes, until the flavors have melded.
6. Using an immersion blender or regular blender, puree the soup until smooth and creamy.
7. Stir in the almond milk, if using, to thin out the soup to your desired consistency.
8. Serve the butternut squash soup hot, garnished with chopped fresh parsley if desired.

Nutrition Facts (per serving):
- Calories: 150
- Total Fat: 4g
- Saturated Fat: 1g
- Cholesterol: 0mg
- Sodium: 360mg
- Total Carbohydrates: 27g
- Dietary Fiber: 6g
- Sugars: 7g
- Protein: 3g

This velvety smooth butternut squash soup is a comforting and nutritious meal. The blend of warming spices complements the natural sweetness of the squash.

Ingredients:

1 medium butternut squash, peeled, seeded, and cubed (about 4 cups)
- 1 tablespoon olive oil
- 1 onion, diced
- 3 cloves garlic, minced
- 4 cups low-sodium vegetable broth
- 1 teaspoon ground cumin
- 1/2 teaspoon ground cinnamon
- 1/4 teaspoon ground nutmeg
- Salt and black pepper to taste
- 2 tablespoons unsweetened almond milk (optional)
- Chopped fresh parsley for garnish (optional)

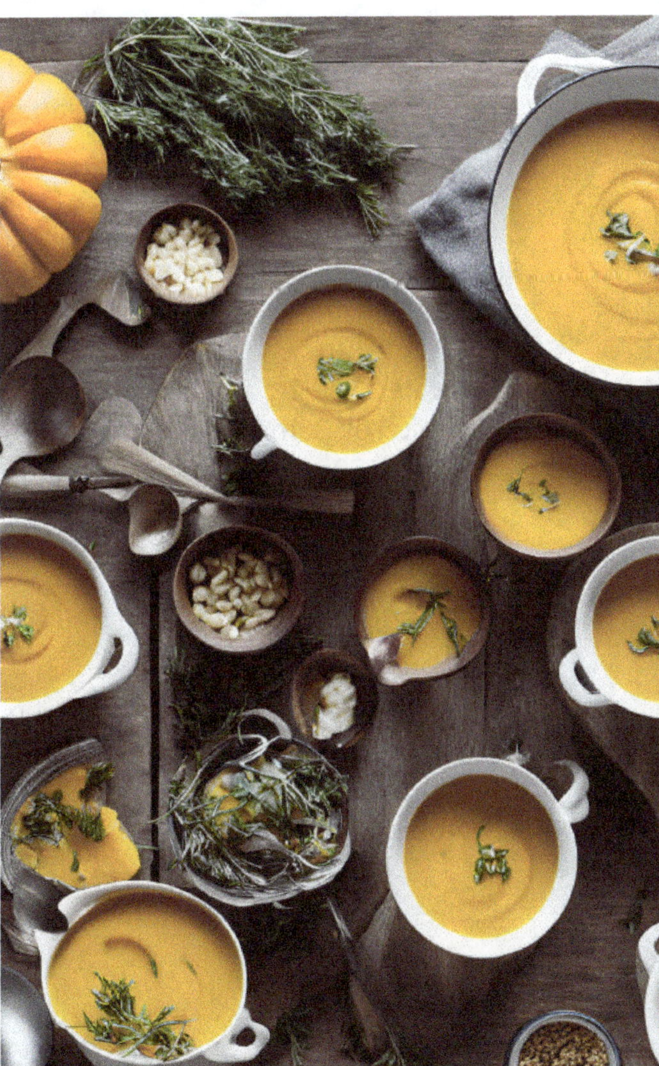

9. Tuna Salad with Mixed Greens

Preparation Time: 10 minutes
Total Time: 10 minutes

Serves: 2

Directions:

1. In a medium bowl, mix together the drained tuna, Greek yogurt, Dijon mustard, lemon juice, red onion, and parsley. Season with salt and pepper.

2. In a large salad bowl, arrange the mixed greens, sliced tomato, and sliced cucumber.

3. In a small bowl, whisk together the olive oil, balsamic vinegar, Dijon mustard, and honey. Season the dressing with salt and pepper.

4. Drizzle the dressing over the salad and toss to coat.

5. Top the salad with the tuna salad mixture.

6. Serve immediately.

Nutrition Facts (per serving):
- Calories: 250
- Total Fat: 12g
- Saturated Fat: 2g
- Cholesterol: 35mg
- Sodium: 550mg
- Total Carbohydrates: 14g
- Dietary Fiber: 4g
- Sugars: 7g
- Protein: 22g

This tuna salad on a bed of mixed greens makes a light and protein-packed lunch or dinner. The tangy dressing complements the flavors of the tuna and vegetables.

Ingredients:

 1 (5 oz) can tuna, drained
- 2 tablespoons plain Greek yogurt
- 1 tablespoon Dijon mustard
- 1 tablespoon lemon juice
- 1 tablespoon finely chopped red onion
- 1 tablespoon chopped fresh parsley
- Salt and pepper to taste
- 4 cups mixed greens (such as spinach, arugula, and kale)
- 1 tomato, sliced
- 1/4 cup sliced cucumber

Dressing:
- 1 tablespoon olive oil
- 1 tablespoon balsamic vinegar
- 1 teaspoon Dijon mustard
- 1 teaspoon honey
- Salt and pepper to taste

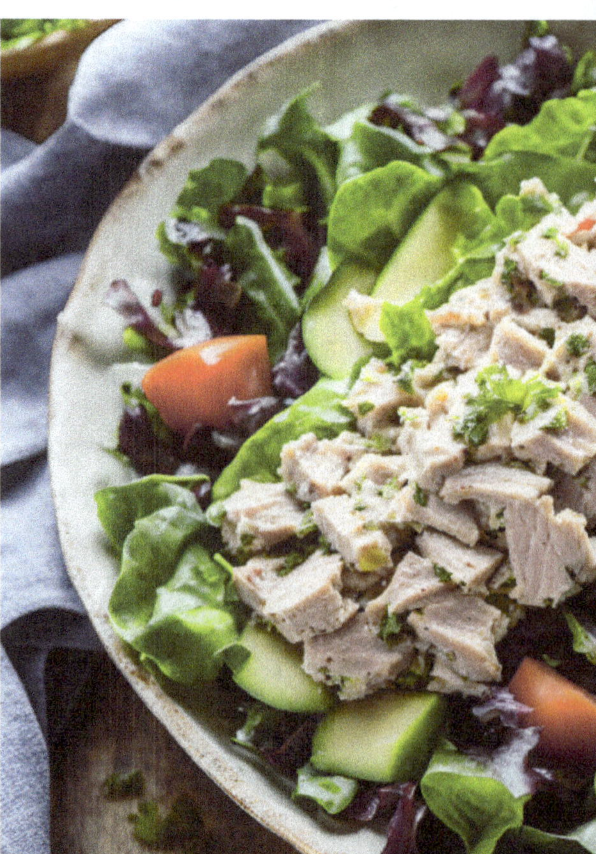

10. Hummus and Veggie Pita Pocket

Preparation Time: 10 minutes
Total Time: 10 minutes

Serves: 1

Directions:

1. Spread the hummus evenly inside the pita bread halves.

2. Layer the sliced cucumber, shredded carrots, and chopped bell pepper inside the pita pockets.

3. Sprinkle the crumbled feta cheese over the top, if using.

4. Season with salt and pepper to taste.

5. Serve immediately.

Nutrition Facts (per serving):
- Calories: 270
- Total Fat: 8g
- Saturated Fat: 2g
- Cholesterol: 5mg
- Sodium: 590mg
- Total Carbohydrates: 41g
- Dietary Fiber: 8g
- Sugars: 6g
- Protein: 10g

This pita pocket is a quick and easy lunch or snack that provides a balance of complex carbohydrates, protein, and fiber. The hummus and vegetables make it a nutritious and satisfying option.

Ingredients:

 1 whole wheat pita bread, halved
- 2 tablespoons hummus
- 1/4 cup sliced cucumber
- 1/4 cup shredded carrots
- 1/4 cup chopped bell pepper
- 1 tablespoon crumbled feta cheese (optional)
- Salt and pepper to taste

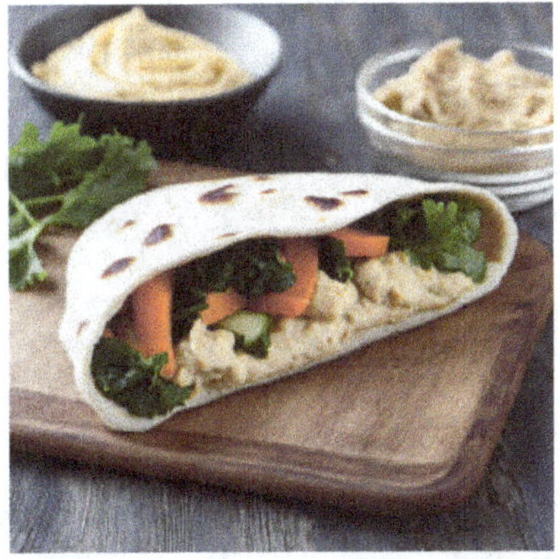

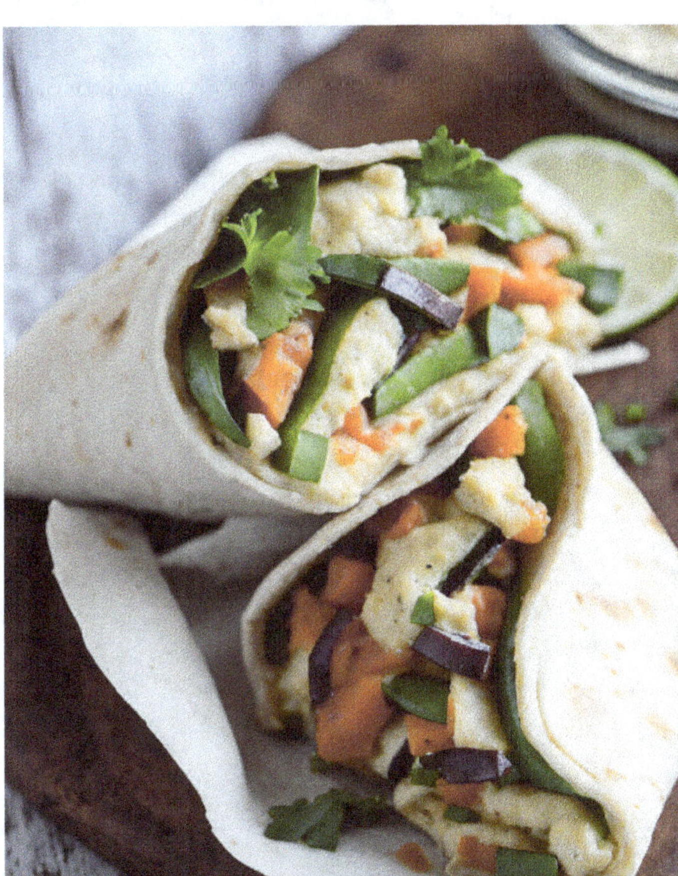

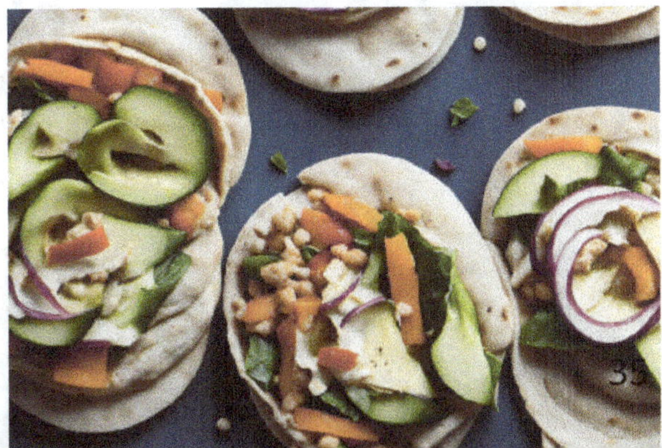

11. Spaghetti Squash with Marinara Sauce

Preparation Time: 15 minutes
Cook Time: 45 minutes
Total Time: 1 hour

Serves: 4

Directions:

1. Preheat the oven to 400°F. Place the spaghetti squash halves cut-side down on a baking sheet. Roast for 40-45 minutes, until tender when pierced with a fork.
2. While the squash is roasting, heat the olive oil in a saucepan over medium heat. Add the diced onion and cook for 5-7 minutes, until translucent.
3. Add the minced garlic and cook for 1 minute, until fragrant.
4. Stir in the crushed tomatoes, tomato paste, dried oregano, and dried basil. Season with salt and black pepper.
5. Reduce the heat to low and let the marinara sauce simmer for 10-15 minutes, stirring occasionally.
6. Once the spaghetti squash is cooked, use a fork to scrape the flesh into strands, creating "spaghetti" noodles.
7. Divide the spaghetti squash noodles among serving plates and top with the warm marinara sauce.
8. Sprinkle the grated Parmesan cheese over the top, if using, and garnish with chopped fresh basil.

Nutrition Facts (per serving):
- Calories: 180
- Total Fat: 5g
- Saturated Fat: 1g
- Cholesterol: 0mg
- Sodium: 390mg
- Total Carbohydrates: 30g
- Dietary Fiber: 6g
- Sugars: 12g
- Protein: 5g

Ingredients:

 1 medium spaghetti squash, halved lengthwise and seeded
- 1 tablespoon olive oil
- 1 onion, diced
- 3 cloves garlic, minced
- 1 (28 oz) can crushed tomatoes
- 2 tablespoons tomato paste
- 1 teaspoon dried oregano
- 1/2 teaspoon dried basil
- Salt and black pepper to taste
- 2 tablespoons grated Parmesan cheese (optional)
- Chopped fresh basil for garnish (optional)

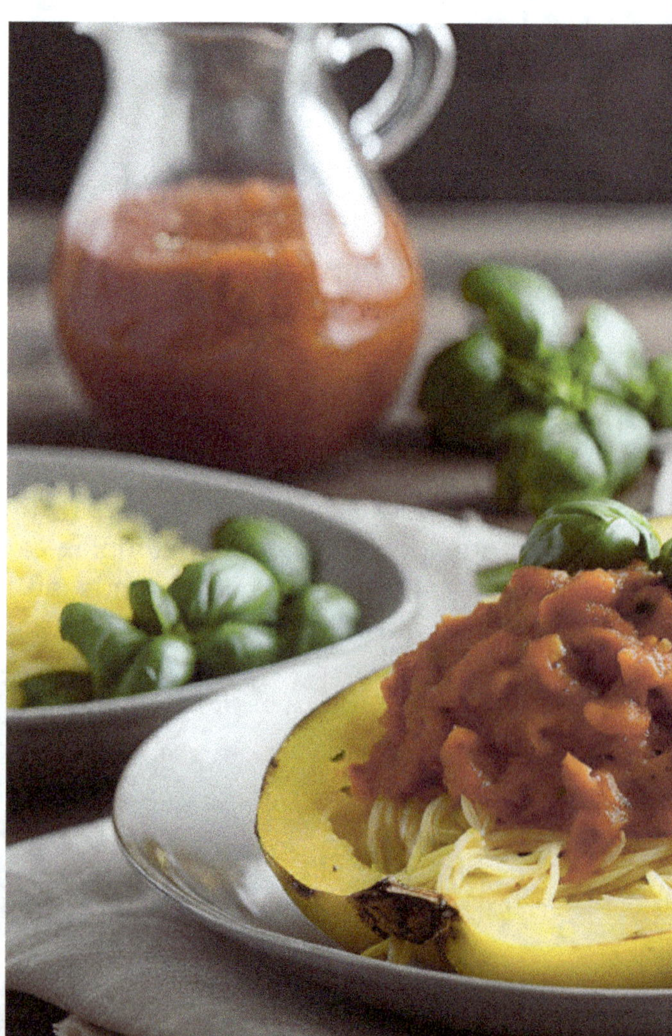

12. Brown Rice and Black Bean Bowl

Preparation Time: 10 minutes
Cook Time: 30 minutes
Total Time: 40 minutes

Serves: 4

Directions:

1. Cook the brown rice according to package instructions.

2. In a large bowl, combine the cooked brown rice, drained and rinsed black beans, diced tomatoes, diced red onion, diced avocado, and chopped fresh cilantro.

3. Drizzle the lime juice over the top and sprinkle with the ground cumin, chili powder, salt, and pepper.

4. Gently toss the ingredients together until well combined.

5. Serve the brown rice and black bean bowl warm or at room temperature.

Nutrition Facts (per serving):
- Calories: 350
- Total Fat: 12g
- Saturated Fat: 2g
- Cholesterol: 0mg
- Sodium: 390mg
- Total Carbohydrates: 52g
- Dietary Fiber: 12g
- Sugars: 4g
- Protein: 11g

This brown rice and black bean bowl is a nutritious and filling vegetarian meal. The combination of whole grains, plant-based protein, healthy fats, and fresh vegetables makes it a well-balanced dish.

Ingredients:

- 1 cup uncooked brown rice
- 1 (15 oz) can black beans, drained and rinsed
- 1 cup diced tomatoes
- 1/2 cup diced red onion
- 1 avocado, diced
- 2 tablespoons chopped fresh cilantro
- 1 tablespoon lime juice
- 1 teaspoon ground cumin
- 1/4 teaspoon chili powder
- Salt and pepper to taste

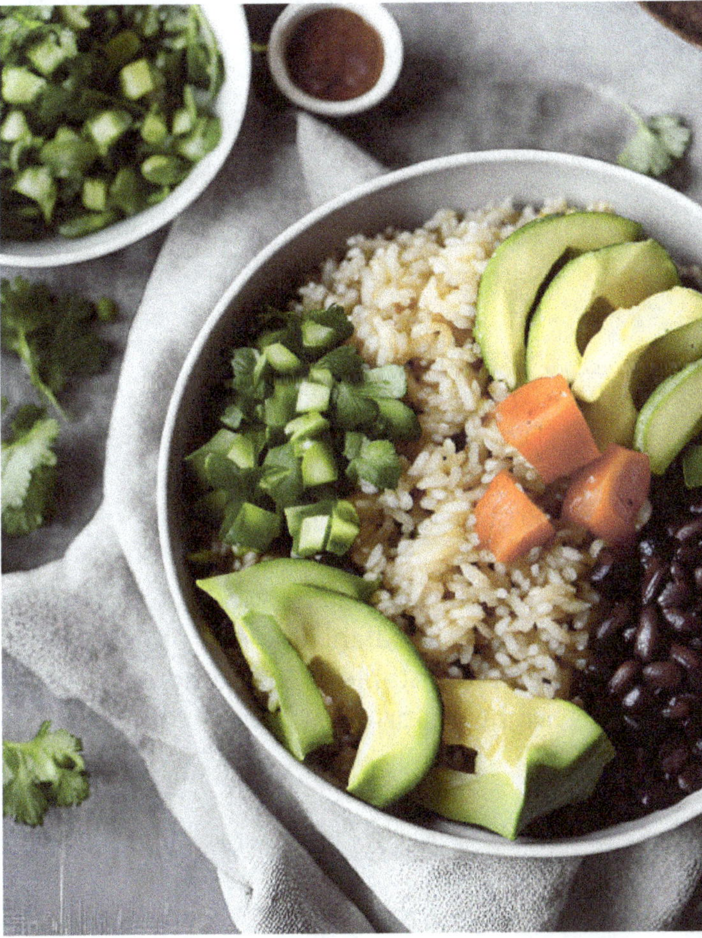

13. Salmon Salad with Lemon Dill Dressing

Preparation Time: 15 minutes
Cook Time: 10 minutes
Total Time: 25 minutes

Serves: 4

Directions:

1. In a large salad bowl, combine the mixed greens, flaked salmon, cherry tomatoes, diced cucumber, and chopped fresh dill.

2. In a small bowl, whisk together the olive oil, lemon juice, Dijon mustard, honey, and chopped fresh dill. Season with salt and pepper.

3. Drizzle the lemon dill dressing over the salad and toss gently to coat.

4. Serve immediately.

Nutrition Facts (per serving):
- Calories: 250
- Total Fat: 14g
- Saturated Fat: 2g
- Cholesterol: 45mg
- Sodium: 450mg
- Total Carbohydrates: 10g
- Dietary Fiber: 3g
- Sugars: 5g
- Protein: 22g

This salmon salad is a nutrient-dense meal that provides a balance of lean protein, healthy fats, and fresh vegetables. The lemon dill dressing adds a bright, flavorful touch.

Ingredients:

For the Salad:
- 4 cups mixed greens (such as spinach, arugula, and romaine)
- 1 (15 oz) can wild-caught salmon, drained and flaked
- 1 cup cherry tomatoes, halved
- 1/2 cup diced cucumber
- 2 tablespoons chopped fresh dill

For the Dressing:
- 2 tablespoons olive oil
- 2 tablespoons lemon juice
- 1 tablespoon Dijon mustard
- 1 teaspoon honey
- 1 teaspoon chopped fresh dill
- Salt and pepper to taste

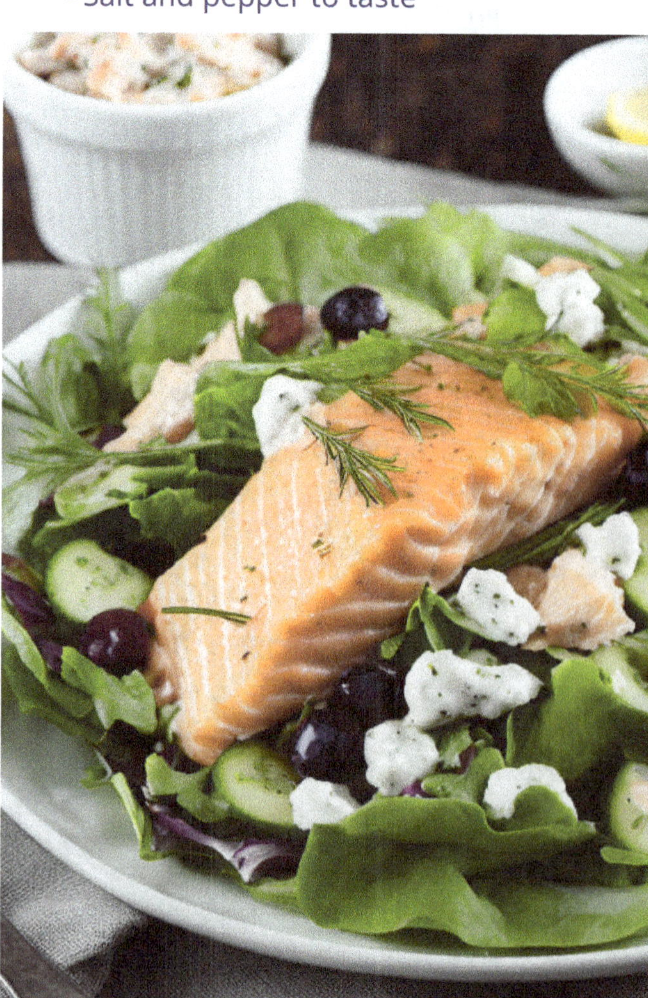

14. Chickpea and Spinach Stew

Preparation Time: 15 minutes
Cook Time: 30 minutes
Total Time: 45 minutes

Serves: 4

Directions:

1. In a large pot or Dutch oven, heat the olive oil over medium heat. Add the diced onion and cook for 5-7 minutes, until translucent.
2. Add the minced garlic, diced carrots, and diced celery. Cook for 3-4 minutes, until the vegetables start to soften.
3. Stir in the ground cumin, smoked paprika, and red pepper flakes (if using). Cook for 1 minute, until fragrant.
4. Add the drained and rinsed chickpeas, diced tomatoes, and vegetable broth. Bring the mixture to a simmer.
5. Reduce the heat to low and let the stew simmer for 20-25 minutes, until the vegetables are tender.
6. Stir in the fresh spinach leaves and cook for 2-3 minutes, until the spinach is wilted.
7. Season the stew with salt and black pepper to taste.
8. Serve the chickpea and spinach stew hot, garnished with chopped fresh parsley if desired.

Nutrition Facts (per serving):
- Calories: 250
- Total Fat: 6g
- Saturated Fat: 1g
- Cholesterol: 0mg
- Sodium: 590mg
- Total Carbohydrates: 38g
- Dietary Fiber: 10g
- Sugars: 8g
- Protein: 11g

Ingredients:

 1 tablespoon olive oil
- 1 onion, diced
- 3 cloves garlic, minced
- 2 carrots, peeled and diced
- 2 celery stalks, diced
- 1 teaspoon ground cumin
- 1/2 teaspoon smoked paprika
- 1/4 teaspoon red pepper flakes (optional)
- 1 (15 oz) can chickpeas, drained and rinsed
- 1 (14.5 oz) can diced tomatoes
- 4 cups low-sodium vegetable broth
- 4 cups fresh spinach leaves
- Salt and black pepper to taste
- Chopped fresh parsley for garnish (optional)

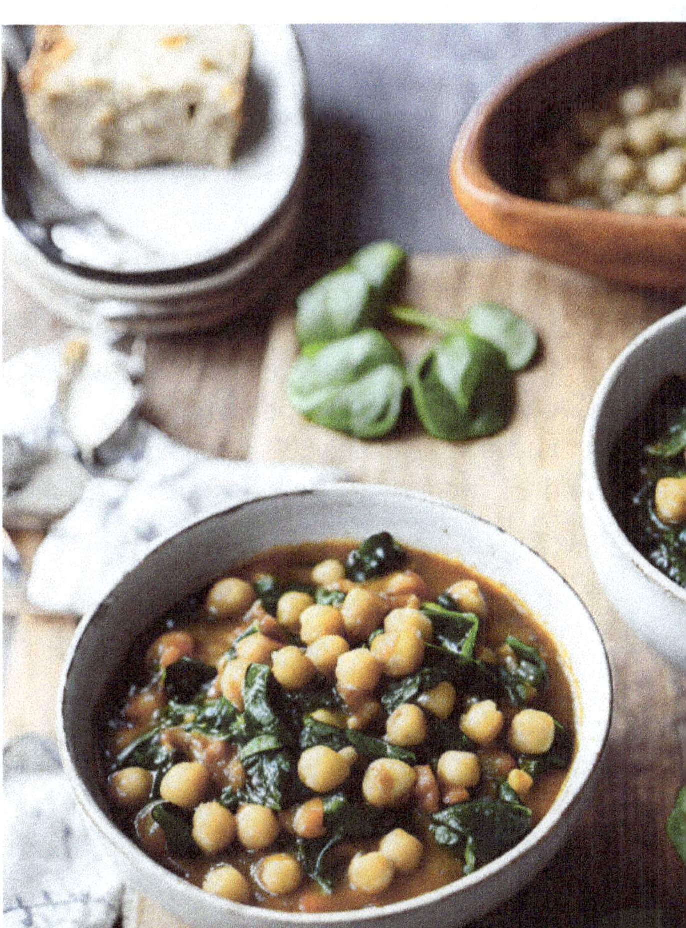

15. Caprese Salad with Fresh Basil

Preparation Time: 10 minutes
Total Time: 10 minutes

Serves: 4

Ingredients:

 8 oz fresh mozzarella cheese, sliced
- 2 medium tomatoes, sliced
- 1/4 cup fresh basil leaves, torn or chopped
- 2 tablespoons balsamic glaze
- 1 tablespoon olive oil
- 1/4 teaspoon salt
- 1/4 teaspoon black pepper

Directions:

1. Arrange the sliced mozzarella cheese and tomatoes on a serving platter or plate.

2. Sprinkle the torn or chopped fresh basil leaves over the top.

3. Drizzle the balsamic glaze and olive oil over the salad.

4. Season with salt and black pepper.

5. Serve immediately.

Nutrition Facts (per serving):
- Calories: 180
- Total Fat: 13g
- Saturated Fat: 6g
- Cholesterol: 30mg
- Sodium: 370mg
- Total Carbohydrates: 7g
- Dietary Fiber: 1g
- Sugars: 6g
- Protein: 11g

This classic Caprese salad showcases the fresh, vibrant flavors of ripe tomatoes, creamy mozzarella, and fragrant basil. The balsamic glaze and olive oil dressing add a delicious finishing touch.

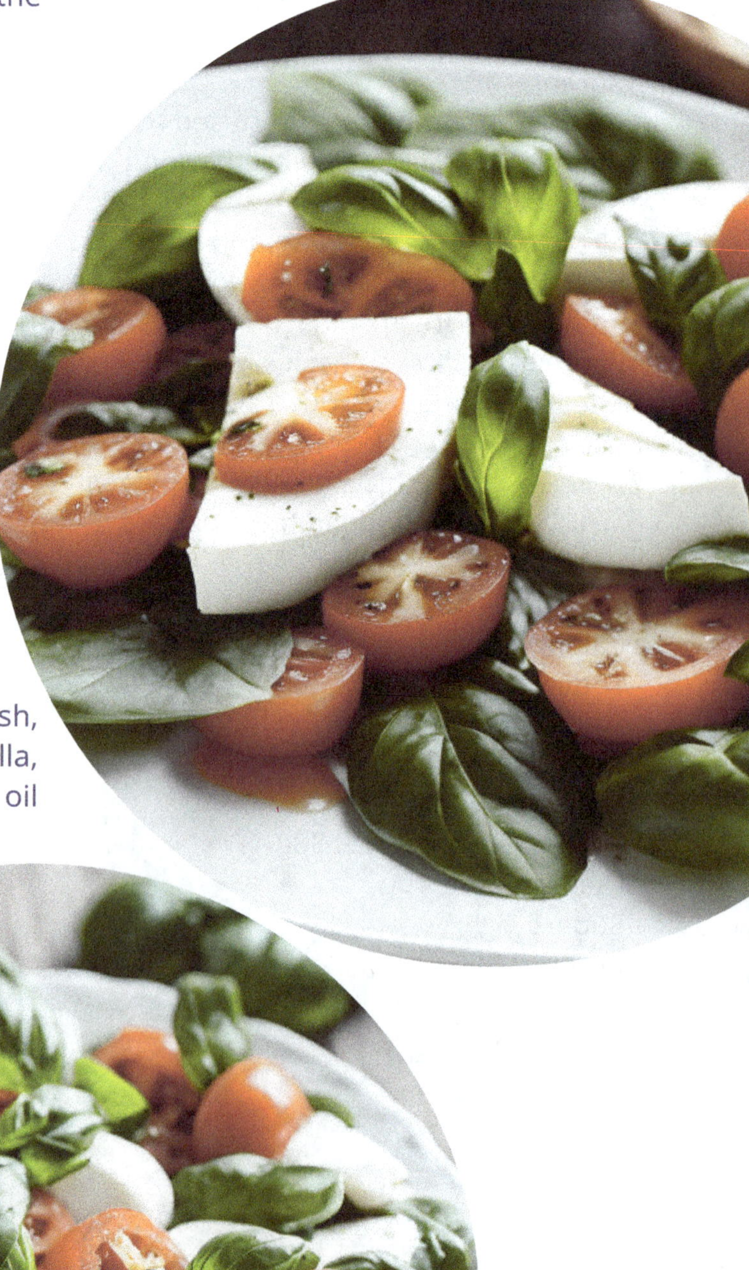

16. Roasted Beet and Goat Cheese Salad

Preparation Time: 15 minutes
Cook Time: 45 minutes
Total Time: 1 hour

Serves: 4

Directions:

1. Preheat the oven to 400°F.

2. Toss the beet cubes with the olive oil and season with salt and pepper.

3. Spread the beets on a baking sheet and roast for 45 minutes, or until tender and caramelized, stirring halfway through.

4. Allow the beets to cool slightly.

5. In a large bowl, combine the roasted beets, mixed greens, crumbled goat cheese, and toasted walnuts.

6. In a small bowl, whisk together the balsamic vinegar and honey. Drizzle the dressing over the salad and toss to coat.

7. Serve immediately.

Nutrition Facts (per serving):
- Calories: 200
- Total Fat: 13g
- Saturated Fat: 5g
- Cholesterol: 15mg
- Sodium: 320mg
- Total Carbohydrates: 16g
- Dietary Fiber: 4g
- Sugars: 10g
- Protein: 8g

Ingredients:

 4 medium beets, peeled and cut into 1-inch cubes
- 2 tablespoons olive oil
- Salt and freshly ground black pepper
- 4 cups mixed greens
- 4 ounces crumbled goat cheese
- 2 tablespoons toasted walnuts
- 2 tablespoons balsamic vinegar
- 1 tablespoon honey

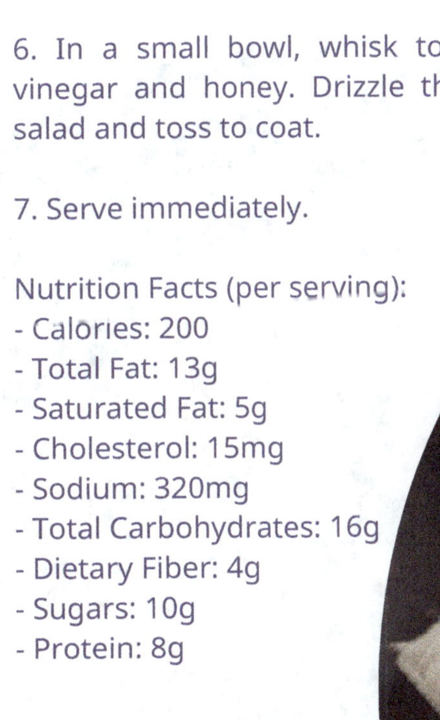

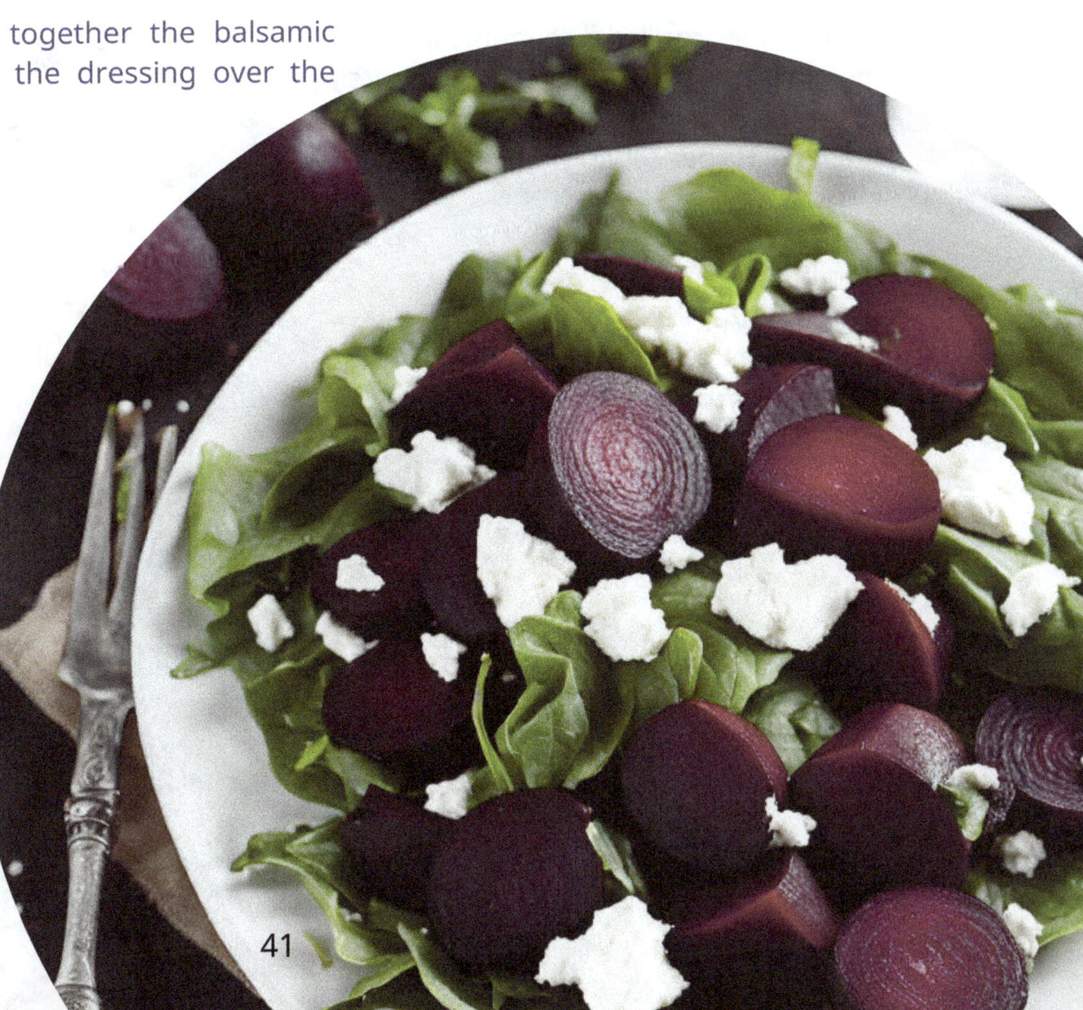

1. Grilled Salmon with Asparagus

Preparation Time: 10 minutes
Cook Time: 15 minutes
Total Time: 25 minutes

Serves: 4

Directions:

1. Preheat grill to medium-high heat.

2. Brush the salmon fillets with olive oil and season with salt and pepper.

3. Grill the salmon for 6-8 minutes per side, or until it flakes easily with a fork.

4. In a large bowl, toss the asparagus with the lemon juice and season with salt and pepper.

5. Grill the asparagus for 5-7 minutes, turning occasionally, until tender-crisp.

6. Serve the grilled salmon and asparagus immediately, garnished with chopped parsley.

Nutrition Facts (per serving):
- Calories: 250
- Total Fat: 14g
- Saturated Fat: 3g
- Cholesterol: 70mg
- Sodium: 650mg
- Total Carbohydrates: 6g
- Dietary Fiber: 3g
- Sugars: 2g
- Protein: 26g

Ingredients:

 4 (6-ounce) salmon fillets
- 1 tablespoon olive oil
- 1 teaspoon salt
- 1/2 teaspoon black pepper
- 1 pound asparagus, trimmed
- 2 tablespoons lemon juice
- 2 tablespoons chopped fresh parsley

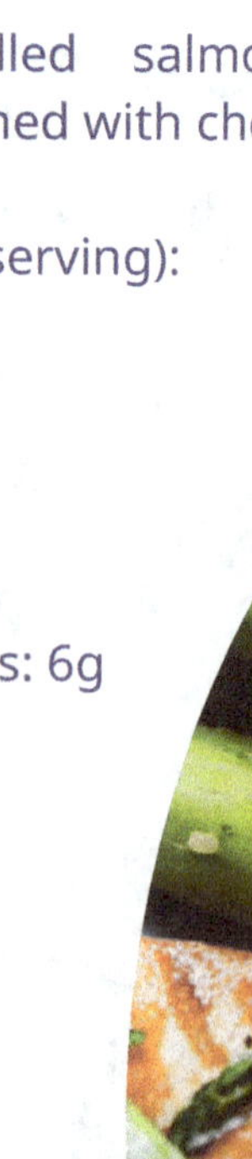
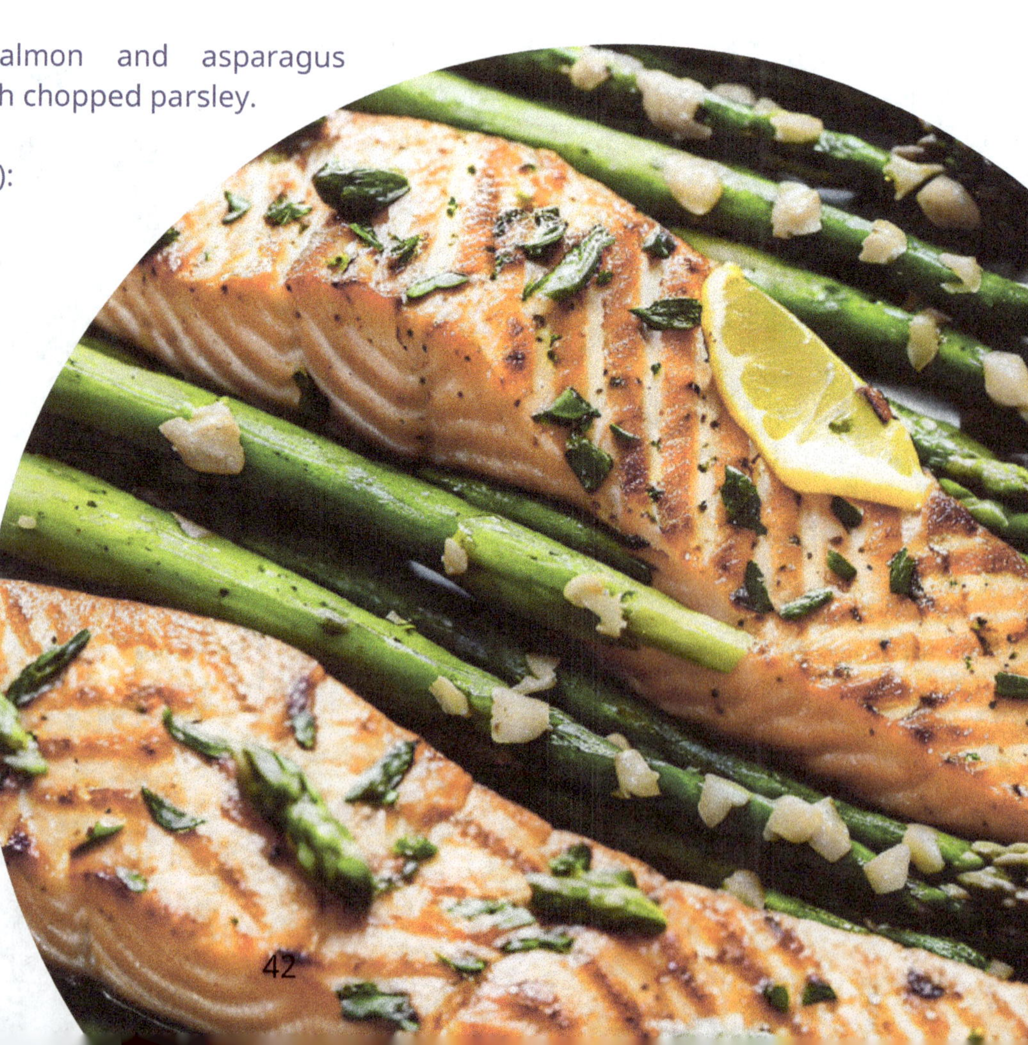

2. Chicken and Broccoli Stir-fry

Preparation Time: 15 minutes
Cook Time: 15 minutes
Total Time: 30 minutes

Serves: 4

Ingredients:

1 pound boneless, skinless chicken breasts, cut into 1-inch pieces
- 2 tablespoons vegetable oil
- 3 cups broccoli florets
- 1 red bell pepper, sliced
- 3 cloves garlic, minced
- 1 tablespoon grated fresh ginger
- 2 tablespoons low-sodium soy sauce
- 1 tablespoon rice vinegar
- 1 teaspoon cornstarch
- 1/4 teaspoon red pepper flakes (optional)
- Cooked rice, for serving

Directions:

1. Heat the vegetable oil in a large skillet or wok over high heat.

2. Add the chicken and stir-fry for 5-7 minutes, until cooked through and no longer pink.

3. Add the broccoli, bell pepper, garlic, and ginger. Stir-fry for 3-4 minutes, until the vegetables are tender-crisp.

4. In a small bowl, whisk together the soy sauce, rice vinegar, and cornstarch. Pour the mixture into the skillet and stir to coat the chicken and vegetables.

5. Bring the sauce to a simmer and cook for 1-2 minutes, until thickened.

6. Remove from heat and stir in the red pepper flakes, if using.

7. Serve the chicken and broccoli stir-fry over cooked rice.

Nutrition Facts (per serving):
- Calories: 280
- Total Fat: 10g
- Saturated Fat: 1.5g
- Cholesterol: 70mg
- Sodium: 480mg
- Total Carbohydrates: 18g
- Dietary Fiber: 4g
- Sugars: 3g
- Protein: 30g

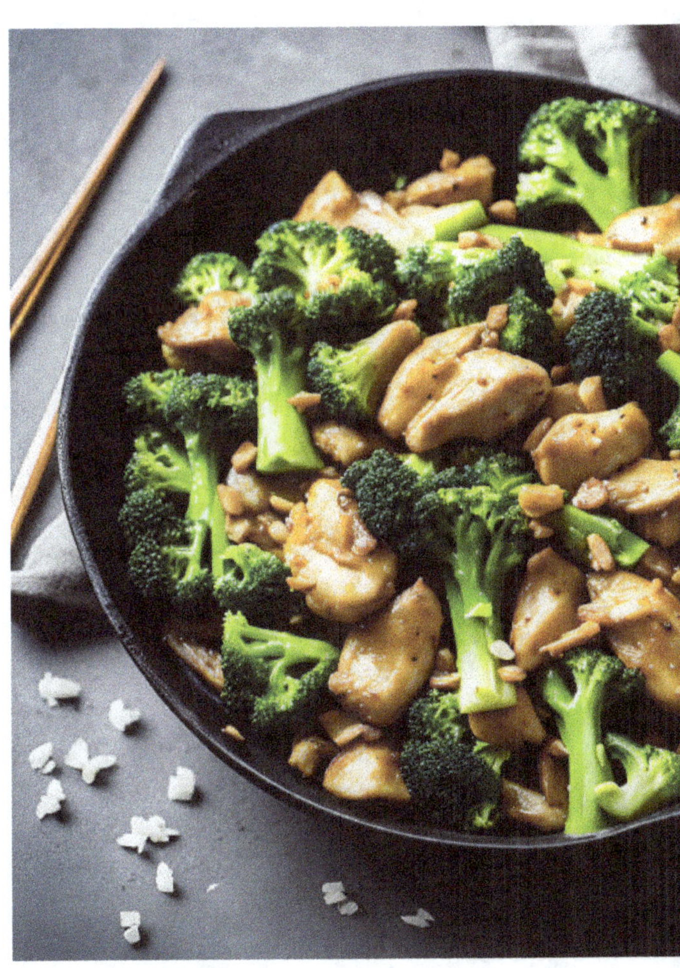

3. Stuffed Bell Peppers with Quinoa and Ground Turkey

Preparation Time: 20 minutes
Cook Time: 40 minutes
Total Time: 1 hour

Serves: 4

Directions:

1. Preheat the oven to 375°F.

2. Place the bell pepper halves in a baking dish and set aside.

3. In a large skillet, cook the ground turkey over medium heat until browned and crumbled, about 5-7 minutes.

4. Add the onion and garlic to the skillet and cook for 2-3 minutes, until fragrant.

5. Stir in the cooked quinoa, diced tomatoes, oregano, basil, and red pepper flakes (if using). Season with salt and black pepper to taste.

6. Spoon the turkey-quinoa mixture into the bell pepper halves, packing it in tightly.

7. Top each stuffed pepper with shredded mozzarella cheese.

8. Bake for 30-40 minutes, or until the peppers are tender and the cheese is melted and bubbly.
9. Serve hot.

Nutrition Facts (per serving):
- Calories: 350
- Total Fat: 16g
- Saturated Fat: 6g
- Cholesterol: 80mg
- Sodium: 550mg
- Total Carbohydrates: 26g
- Dietary Fiber: 6g
- Sugars: 8g
- Protein: 29g

Ingredients:

 4 large bell peppers, halved and seeded
- 1 pound ground turkey
- 1 cup cooked quinoa
- 1 small onion, diced
- 2 cloves garlic, minced
- 1 (14.5 oz) can diced tomatoes
- 1 teaspoon dried oregano
- 1/2 teaspoon dried basil
- 1/4 teaspoon red pepper flakes (optional)
- Salt and black pepper, to taste
- 1 cup shredded mozzarella cheese

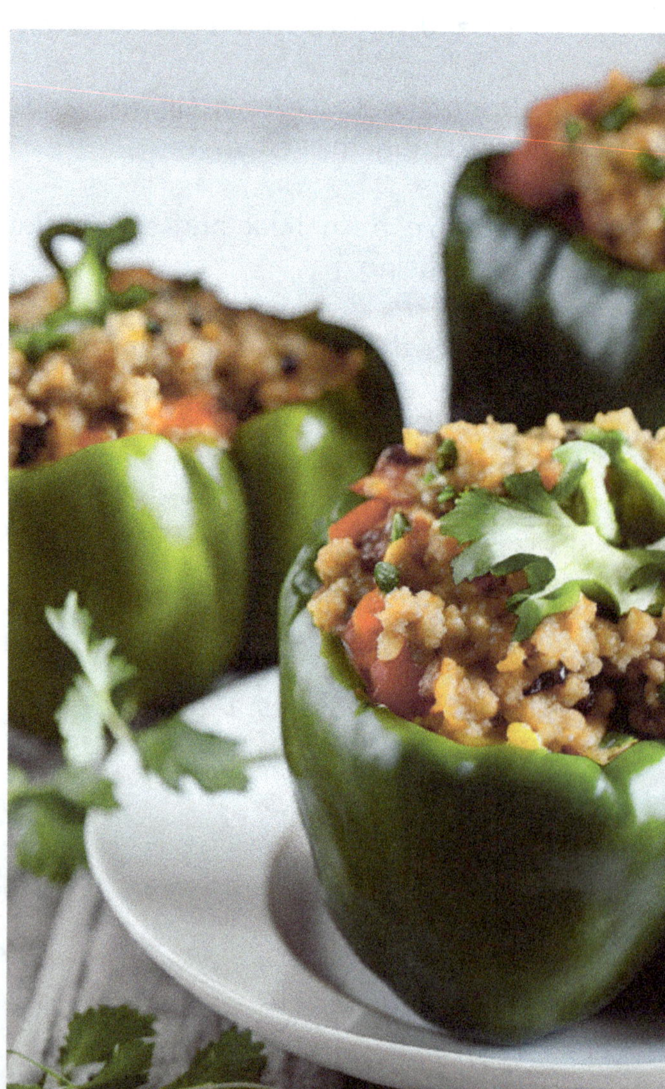

4. Vegetable and Tofu Curry

Preparation Time: 20 minutes
Cook Time: 30 minutes
Total Time: 50 minutes

Serves: 4

Directions:

1. In a large skillet or wok, heat the vegetable oil over medium-high heat. Add the cubed tofu and cook, stirring occasionally, until lightly browned on all sides, about 5-7 minutes. Transfer the tofu to a plate and set aside.

2. In the same skillet, add the onion and cook for 3-4 minutes, until translucent. Add the garlic and ginger and cook for 1 minute, until fragrant.

3. Stir in the curry powder, cumin, coriander, and cayenne (if using). Cook for 1 minute to toast the spices.

4. Add the carrots, cauliflower, and potatoes to the skillet. Pour in the coconut milk and vegetable broth. Bring the mixture to a simmer and cook for 15-20 minutes, or until the vegetables are tender.

5. Stir in the soy sauce and the reserved tofu. Season with salt and black pepper to taste.

6. Serve the vegetable and tofu curry over cooked rice, garnished with chopped cilantro.

Nutrition Facts (per serving):
- Calories: 350
- Total Fat: 22g
- Saturated Fat: 13g
- Cholesterol: 0mg
- Sodium: 650mg
- Total Carbohydrates: 30g
- Dietary Fiber: 6g
- Sugars: 6g
- Protein: 16g

Ingredients:

 1 block (14 oz) extra-firm tofu, cubed
- 2 tablespoons vegetable oil
- 1 onion, diced
- 3 cloves garlic, minced
- 1 tablespoon grated fresh ginger
- 2 tablespoons curry powder
- 1 teaspoon ground cumin
- 1/2 teaspoon ground coriander
- 1/4 teaspoon cayenne pepper (optional)
- 1 cup diced carrots
- 1 cup diced cauliflower
- 1 cup diced potatoes
- 1 (13.5 oz) can coconut milk
- 1 cup vegetable broth
- 1 tablespoon soy sauce
- Salt and black pepper, to taste
- Chopped cilantro, for garnish
- Cooked rice, for serving

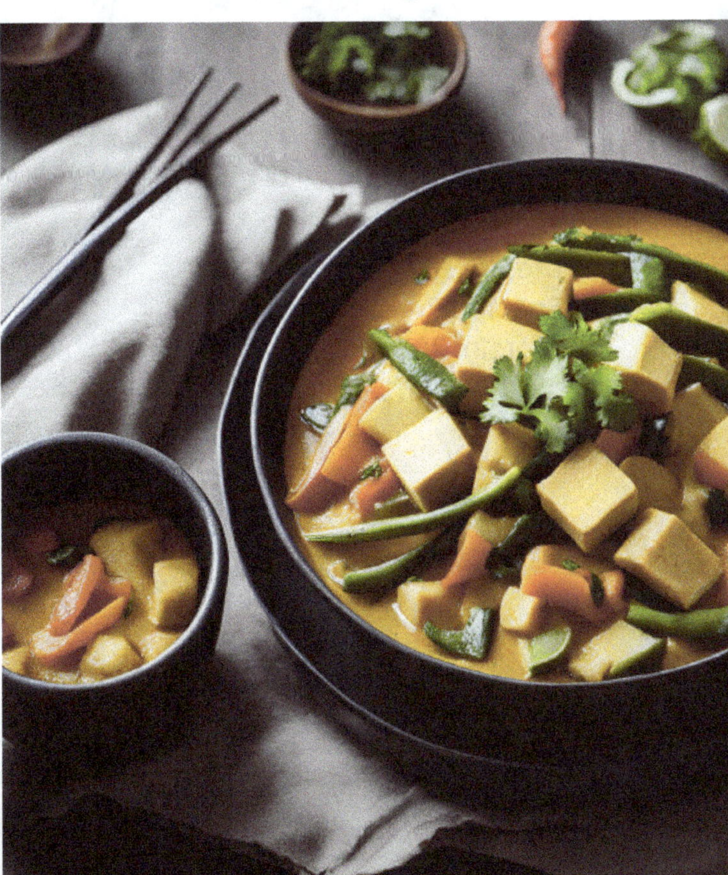

5. Baked Cod with Lemon and Dill

Preparation Time: 10 minutes
Cook Time: 20 minutes
Total Time: 30 minutes

Serves: 4

Directions:

1. Preheat the oven to 400°F.

2. Place the cod fillets in a baking dish.

3. In a small bowl, whisk together the olive oil, lemon juice, dill, lemon zest, salt, and pepper.

4. Drizzle the lemon-dill mixture over the cod fillets, making sure to evenly coat the fish.

5. Bake for 18-20 minutes, or until the cod is opaque and flakes easily with a fork.

6. Serve the baked cod immediately, garnished with additional fresh dill if desired.

Nutrition Facts (per serving):
- Calories: 180
- Total Fat: 7g
- Saturated Fat: 1g
- Cholesterol: 70mg
- Sodium: 420mg
- Total Carbohydrates: 0g
- Dietary Fiber: 0g
- Sugars: 0g
- Protein: 26g

Ingredients:

 4 (6-ounce) cod fillets
- 2 tablespoons olive oil
- 2 tablespoons lemon juice
- 2 tablespoons chopped fresh dill
- 1 teaspoon grated lemon zest
- 1/2 teaspoon salt
- 1/4 teaspoon black pepper

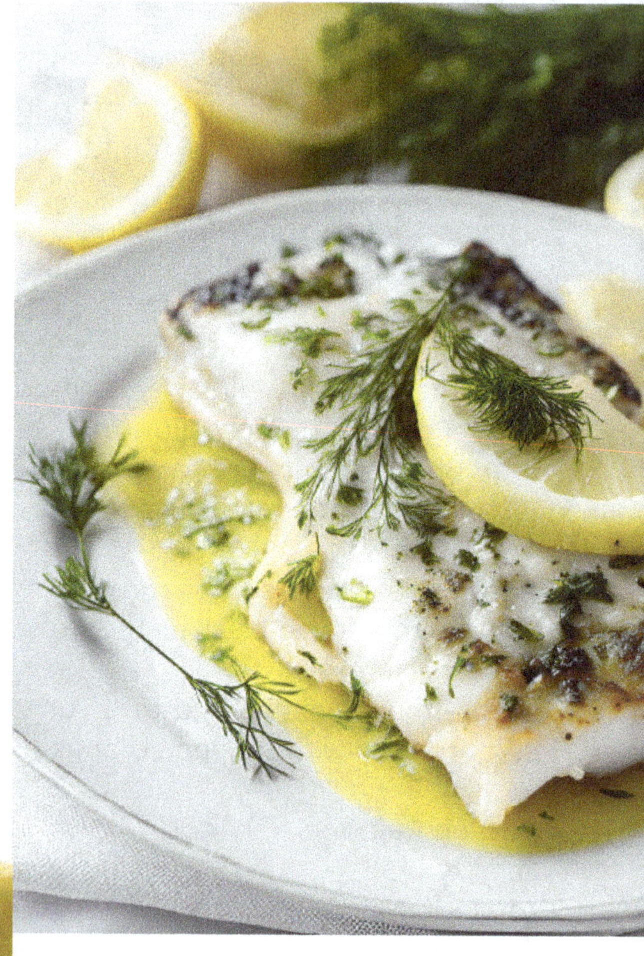

6. Beef and Vegetable Kebabs

Preparation Time: 20 minutes
Cook Time: 15 minutes
Total Time: 35 minutes

Serves: 4

Directions:

1. Preheat grill to medium-high heat.

2. In a large bowl, combine the beef cubes, bell pepper pieces, onion pieces, and mushrooms.

3. In a small bowl, whisk together the olive oil, balsamic vinegar, oregano, salt, and black pepper.

4. Pour the marinade over the beef and vegetables and toss to coat evenly.

5. Thread the marinated beef and vegetables onto skewers, alternating the ingredients.

6. Grill the kebabs for 12-15 minutes, turning occasionally, until the beef is cooked through and the vegetables are tender.

7. Serve the beef and vegetable kebabs immediately.

Nutrition Facts (per serving):
- Calories: 280
- Total Fat: 14g
- Saturated Fat: 3.5g
- Cholesterol: 65mg
- Sodium: 450mg
- Total Carbohydrates: 14g
- Dietary Fiber: 3g
- Sugars: 8g
- Protein: 26g

Ingredients:

 1 pound beef sirloin, cut into 1-inch cubes
- 1 red bell pepper, cut into 1-inch pieces
- 1 yellow bell pepper, cut into 1-inch pieces
- 1 red onion, cut into 1-inch pieces
- 8 ounces mushrooms, halved
- 2 tablespoons olive oil
- 2 tablespoons balsamic vinegar
- 1 teaspoon dried oregano
- 1/2 teaspoon salt
- 1/4 teaspoon black pepper

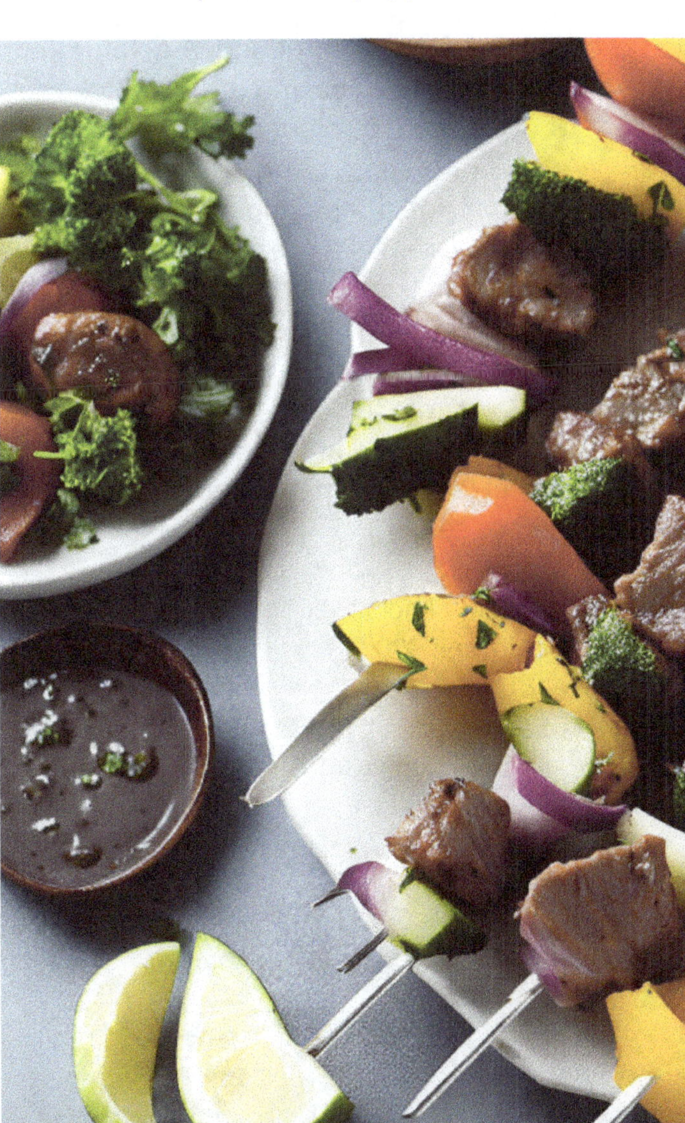

7. Lentil and Vegetable Shepherd's Pie

Preparation Time: 30 minutes
Cook Time: 45 minutes
Total Time: 1 hour 15 minutes

Serves: 6

Directions:

1. Preheat the oven to 375°F.
2. In a medium saucepan, combine the lentils and vegetable broth. Bring to a boil, then reduce heat and simmer for 20-25 minutes, until the lentils are tender. Drain any excess liquid and set aside.
3. In a large skillet, heat the olive oil over medium heat. Add the onion and sauté for 5 minutes, until translucent. Add the garlic, carrots, and celery, and sauté for another 5 minutes.
4. Stir in the cooked lentils, frozen peas, thyme, rosemary, and season with salt and black pepper to taste.
5. Transfer the lentil and vegetable mixture to a 9-inch pie dish or baking dish.
6. In a medium saucepan, cover the potato cubes with water and bring to a boil. Reduce heat and simmer for 15-20 minutes, until the potatoes are tender. Drain the potatoes and mash them with the almond milk and butter. Season with salt.
7. Spread the mashed potatoes over the lentil and vegetable mixture, smoothing the top.
8. Bake for 30-35 minutes, until the potatoes are lightly browned and the filling is bubbling.
9. Let the shepherd's pie cool for 5-10 minutes before serving.

Nutrition Facts (per serving):
- Calories: 320
- Total Fat: 9g
- Saturated Fat: 3g
- Cholesterol: 10mg
- Sodium: 650mg
- Total Carbohydrates: 48g
- Dietary Fiber: 12g
- Sugars: 6g
- Protein: 13g

Ingredients:

For the Filling:
- 1 cup brown lentils, rinsed
- 3 cups vegetable broth
- 1 tablespoon olive oil
- 1 onion, diced
- 3 cloves garlic, minced
- 2 carrots, diced
- 2 celery stalks, diced
- 1 cup frozen peas
- 1 teaspoon dried thyme
- 1 teaspoon dried rosemary
- Salt and black pepper, to taste

For the Topping:
- 3 medium potatoes, peeled and cut into 1-inch cubes
- 1/4 cup unsweetened almond milk
- 2 tablespoons butter
- 1/2 teaspoon salt

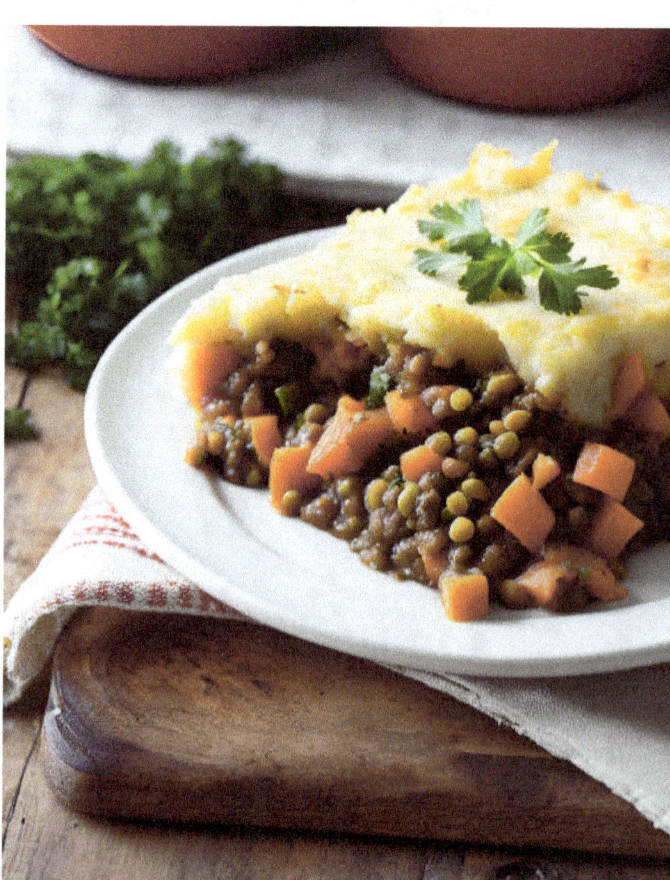

8. Spaghetti with Zucchini Noodles and Pesto

Preparation Time: 20 minutes
Cook Time: 15 minutes
Total Time: 35 minutes

Serves: 4

Directions:

1. Bring a large pot of salted water to a boil. Cook the spaghetti according to package instructions, until al dente. Drain and set aside.

2. In a food processor, combine the basil, garlic, pine nuts, Parmesan, olive oil, salt, and pepper. Pulse until a smooth pesto forms.

3. In a large skillet, heat the spiralized or julienned zucchini over medium heat for 3-5 minutes, until tender but still crisp.

4. Add the cooked spaghetti and pesto to the skillet with the zucchini noodles. Toss to combine and coat the noodles evenly with the pesto.

5. Serve the spaghetti with zucchini noodles and pesto immediately.

Nutrition Facts (per serving):
- Calories: 320
- Total Fat: 16g
- Saturated Fat: 3g
- Cholesterol: 5mg
- Sodium: 380mg
- Total Carbohydrates: 35g
- Dietary Fiber: 5g
- Sugars: 4g
- Protein: 12g

Ingredients:

  3 medium zucchini, spiralized or julienned
- 8 ounces whole wheat spaghetti
- 1 cup fresh basil leaves
- 2 cloves garlic
- 1/4 cup pine nuts
- 1/4 cup grated Parmesan cheese
- 2 tablespoons olive oil
- 1/4 teaspoon salt
- 1/4 teaspoon black pepper

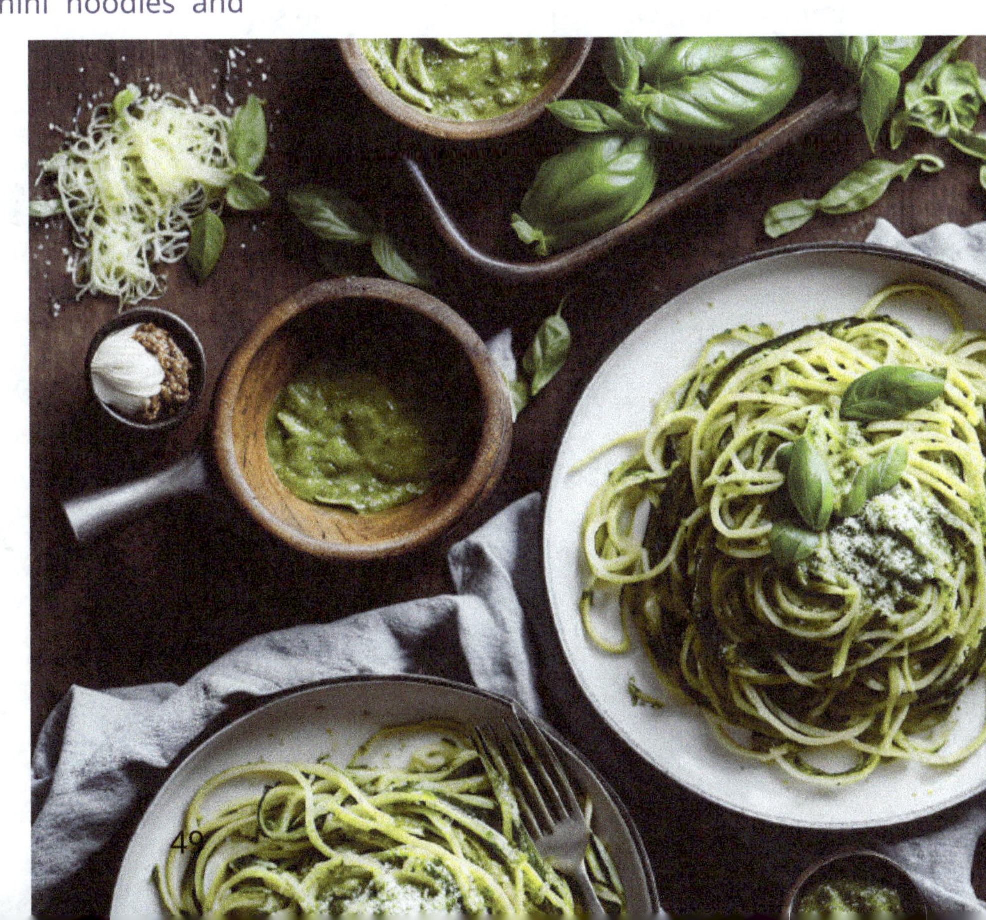

9. Roasted Chicken with Brussels Sprouts

Preparation Time: 15 minutes
Cook Time: 45 minutes
Total Time: 1 hour

Serves: 4

Ingredients:

 1 whole chicken (3-4 pounds), cut into 8 pieces (breasts, thighs, drumsticks, wings)
- 1 pound Brussels sprouts, trimmed and halved
- 2 tablespoons olive oil
- 1 teaspoon salt
- 1/2 teaspoon black pepper
- 1 lemon, cut into wedges (for serving)

Directions:

1. Preheat the oven to 400°F.

2. Arrange the chicken pieces and Brussels sprouts on a large baking sheet. Drizzle with the olive oil and season with salt and pepper. Toss to coat everything evenly.

3. Roast for 40-45 minutes, or until the chicken is cooked through (internal temperature reaches 165°F) and the Brussels sprouts are tender and caramelized.

4. Remove the baking sheet from the oven and let the chicken rest for 5 minutes.

5. Serve the roasted chicken and Brussels sprouts immediately, with lemon wedges on the side.

Nutrition Facts (per serving):
- Calories: 400
- Total Fat: 22g
- Saturated Fat: 5g
- Cholesterol: 135mg
- Sodium: 750mg
- Total Carbohydrates: 14g
- Dietary Fiber: 5g
- Sugars: 3g
- Protein: 40g

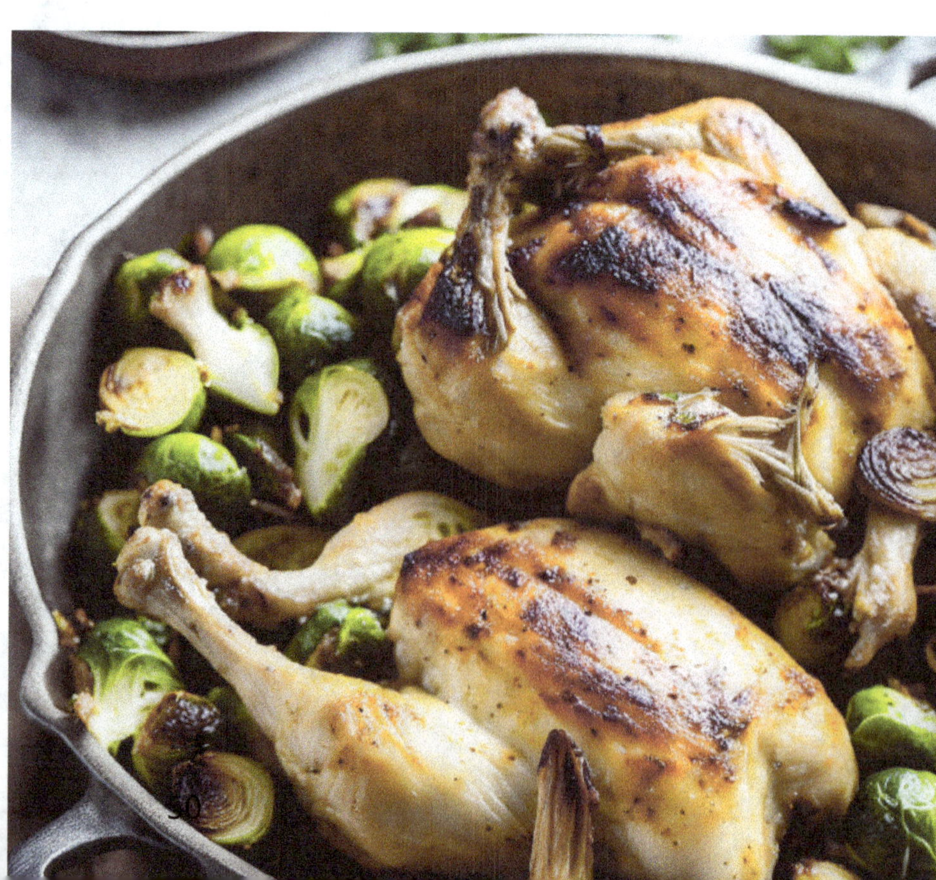

10. Shrimp and Avocado Salad

Preparation Time: 15 minutes
Cook Time: 5 minutes
Total Time: 20 minutes

Serves: 4

Directions:

1. In a large bowl, combine the cooked shrimp, diced avocados, cherry tomatoes, red onion, and chopped cilantro.

2. In a small bowl, whisk together the lime juice, olive oil, salt, and black pepper.

3. Pour the dressing over the shrimp and avocado mixture and gently toss to coat.

4. Serve the shrimp and avocado salad immediately, or refrigerate until ready to serve.

Nutrition Facts (per serving):
- Calories: 260
- Total Fat: 16g
- Saturated Fat: 2.5g
- Cholesterol: 170mg
- Sodium: 550mg
- Total Carbohydrates: 12g
- Dietary Fiber: 6g
- Sugars: 3g
- Protein: 20g

Ingredients:

 1 pound cooked shrimp, peeled and deveined
- 2 avocados, diced
- 1 cup cherry tomatoes, halved
- 1/2 red onion, thinly sliced
- 2 tablespoons chopped fresh cilantro
- 2 tablespoons lime juice
- 1 tablespoon olive oil
- 1/4 teaspoon salt
- 1/4 teaspoon black pepper

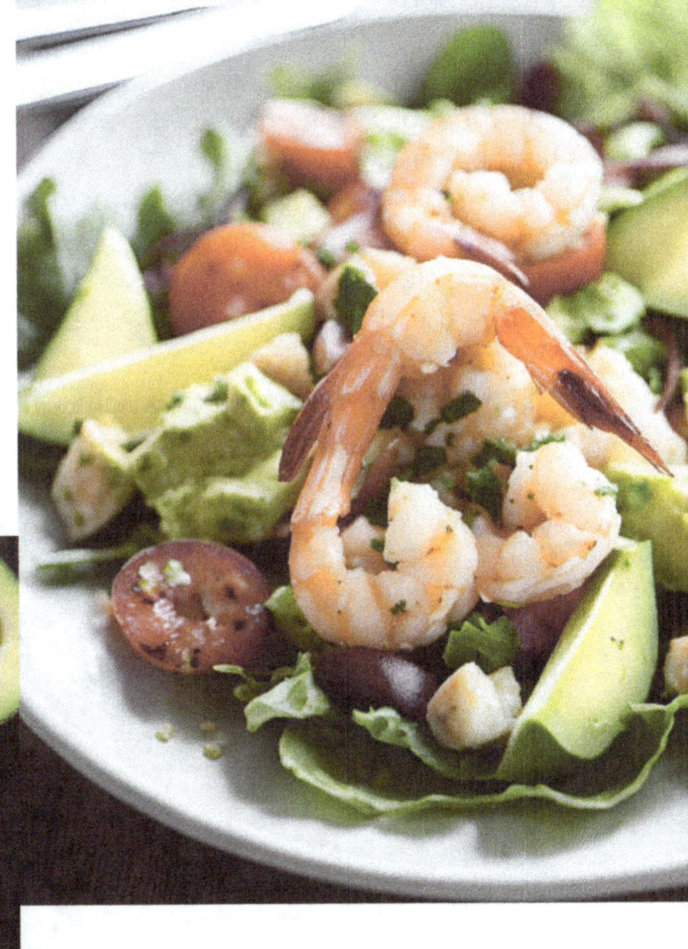

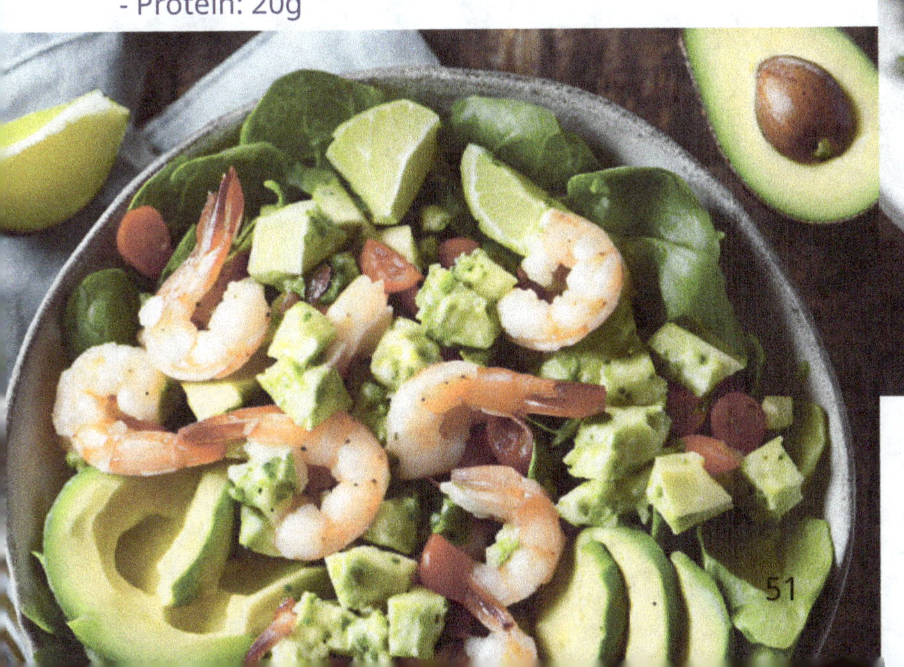

11. Pork Tenderloin with Apple Slaw

Preparation Time: 20 minutes
Cook Time: 25 minutes
Total Time: 45 minutes

Serves: 4

Directions:

1. Preheat the oven to 400°F.
2. Season the pork tenderloin with the salt and black pepper.
3. Heat the 1 tablespoon of olive oil in a large oven-safe skillet over medium-high heat. Sear the pork tenderloin on all sides until browned, about 2-3 minutes per side.
4. Transfer the skillet to the preheated oven and roast the pork for 15-20 minutes, or until it reaches an internal temperature of 145°F.
5. Remove the pork from the oven and let it rest for 5 minutes before slicing.
6. In a large bowl, combine the shredded green and red cabbage, julienned or grated apples, and chopped parsley.
7. In a small bowl, whisk together the apple cider vinegar, Dijon mustard, honey, 2 tablespoons of olive oil, salt, and black pepper.
8. Pour the dressing over the cabbage and apple mixture and toss to coat.
9. Serve the sliced pork tenderloin with the apple slaw on the side.

Nutrition Facts (per serving):
- Calories: 320
- Total Fat: 14g
- Saturated Fat: 2.5g
- Cholesterol: 80mg
- Sodium: 650mg
- Total Carbohydrates: 20g
- Dietary Fiber: 4g
- Sugars: 14g
- Protein: 30g

Ingredients:

or the Pork Tenderloin:
- 1 pound pork tenderloin
- 1 tablespoon olive oil
- 1 teaspoon salt
- 1/2 teaspoon black pepper

For the Apple Slaw:
- 2 cups shredded green cabbage
- 1 cup shredded red cabbage
- 2 apples, julienned or grated
- 1/4 cup chopped fresh parsley
- 2 tablespoons apple cider vinegar
- 1 tablespoon Dijon mustard
- 1 tablespoon honey
- 2 tablespoons olive oil
- 1/4 teaspoon salt
- 1/4 teaspoon black pepper

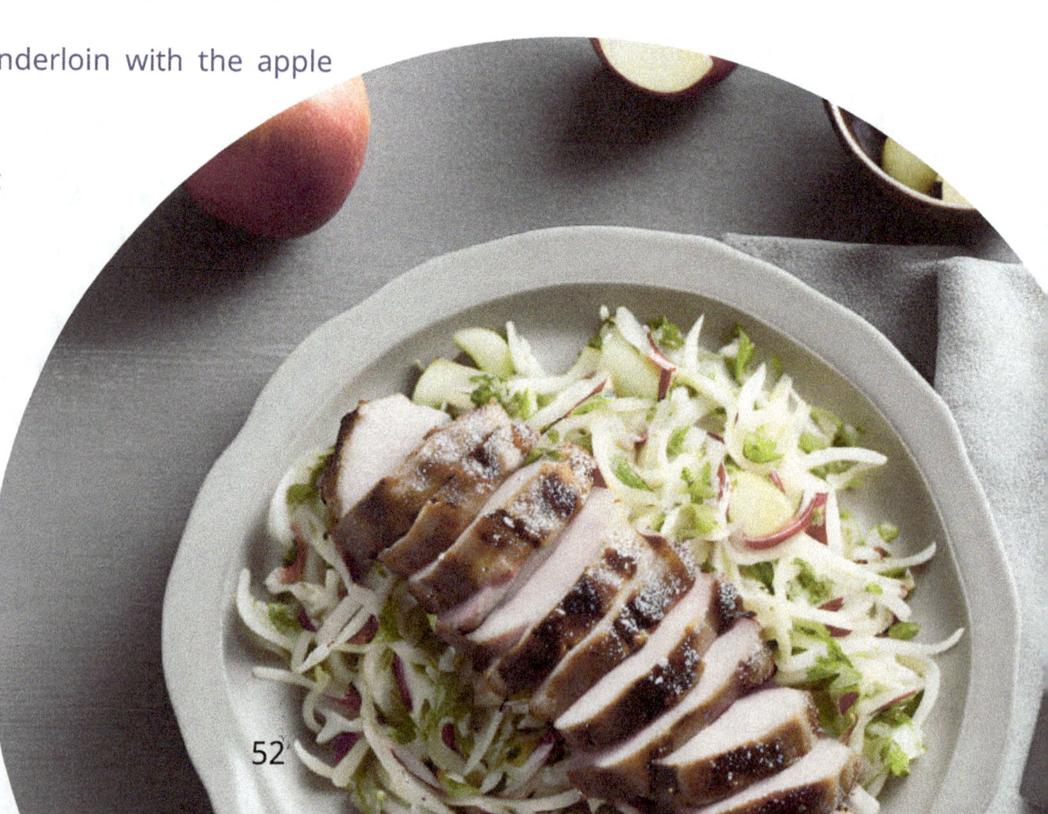

12. Vegetable Paella

Preparation Time: 20 minutes
Cook Time: 40 minutes
Total Time: 1 hour

Serves: 4

Directions:

1. Heat the olive oil in a large, shallow pan or paella pan over medium heat.
2. Add the diced onion and sauté for 3-4 minutes, until translucent.
3. Stir in the minced garlic and diced bell pepper. Cook for 2-3 minutes, until fragrant.
4. Add the uncooked rice, smoked paprika, and saffron (if using). Stir to coat the rice with the spices and oil.
5. Pour in the vegetable broth and diced tomatoes. Bring the mixture to a simmer.
6. Reduce heat to low, cover the pan, and let the rice cook for 15 minutes, without stirring.
7. After 15 minutes, add the frozen peas, sliced mushrooms, and diced zucchini. Cover and cook for an additional 10-15 minutes, or until the rice is tender and the vegetables are cooked through.
8. Season the paella with salt and black pepper to taste.
9. Serve the vegetable paella hot, garnished with chopped parsley.

Nutrition Facts (per serving):
- Calories: 320
- Total Fat: 8g
- Saturated Fat: 1g
- Cholesterol: 0mg
- Sodium: 550mg
- Total Carbohydrates: 52g
- Dietary Fiber: 7g
- Sugars: 7g
- Protein: 9g

Ingredients:

 2 tablespoons olive oil
- 1 onion, diced
- 3 cloves garlic, minced
- 1 red bell pepper, diced
- 1 cup uncooked short-grain rice (such as Arborio)
- 1 teaspoon smoked paprika
- 1/2 teaspoon saffron threads (optional)
- 1 cup vegetable broth
- 1 (14.5 oz) can diced tomatoes
- 1 cup frozen peas
- 1 cup sliced mushrooms
- 1 zucchini, diced
- Salt and black pepper, to taste
- Chopped parsley, for garnish

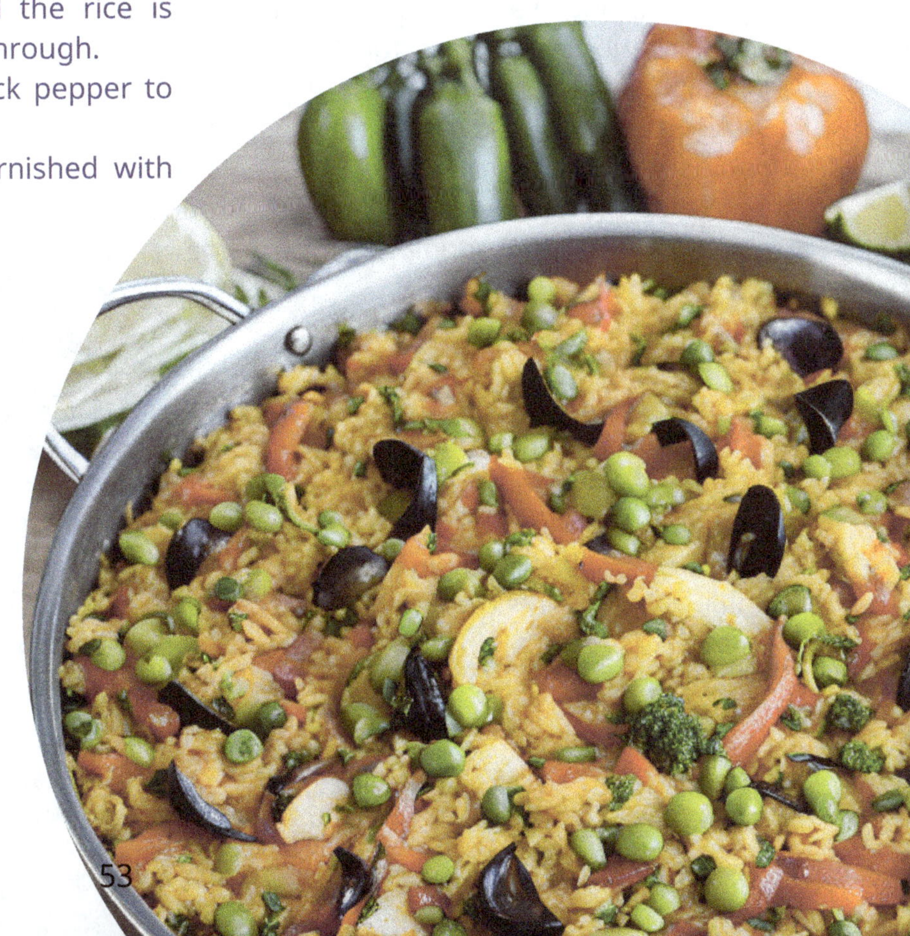

13. Turkey Meatballs with Tomato Sauce

Preparation Time: 20 minutes
Cook Time: 30 minutes
Total Time: 50 minutes

Serves: 4

Directions:

1. Preheat the oven to 400°F.
2. In a large bowl, combine all the meatball ingredients and mix well until fully incorporated.
3. Roll the mixture into 1-inch meatballs and place them on a baking sheet lined with parchment paper.
4. Bake the meatballs for 20-25 minutes, or until cooked through.
5. While the meatballs are baking, heat the olive oil in a large saucepan over medium heat.
6. Add the diced onion and sauté for 3-4 minutes, until translucent.
7. Stir in the minced garlic and cook for 1 minute, until fragrant.
8. Add the crushed tomatoes, tomato paste, dried basil, salt, and black pepper. Bring the sauce to a simmer and let it cook for 10 minutes, stirring occasionally.
9. Add the cooked meatballs to the tomato sauce and gently stir to coat.
10. Serve the turkey meatballs with tomato sauce over pasta, zucchini noodles, or with a side salad.

Nutrition Facts (per serving):
- Calories: 350
- Total Fat: 15g
- Saturated Fat: 4g
- Cholesterol: 100mg
- Sodium: 850mg
- Total Carbohydrates: 28g
- Dietary Fiber: 5g
- Sugars: 10g
- Protein: 28g

Ingredients:

or the Meatballs:
- 1 pound ground turkey
- 1/2 cup breadcrumbs
- 1/4 cup grated Parmesan cheese
- 1 egg
- 2 cloves garlic, minced
- 1 teaspoon dried oregano
- 1/2 teaspoon salt
- 1/4 teaspoon black pepper

For the Tomato Sauce:
- 1 tablespoon olive oil
- 1 onion, diced
- 3 cloves garlic, minced
- 1 (28 oz) can crushed tomatoes
- 2 tablespoons tomato paste
- 1 teaspoon dried basil
- 1/2 teaspoon salt
- 1/4 teaspoon black pepper

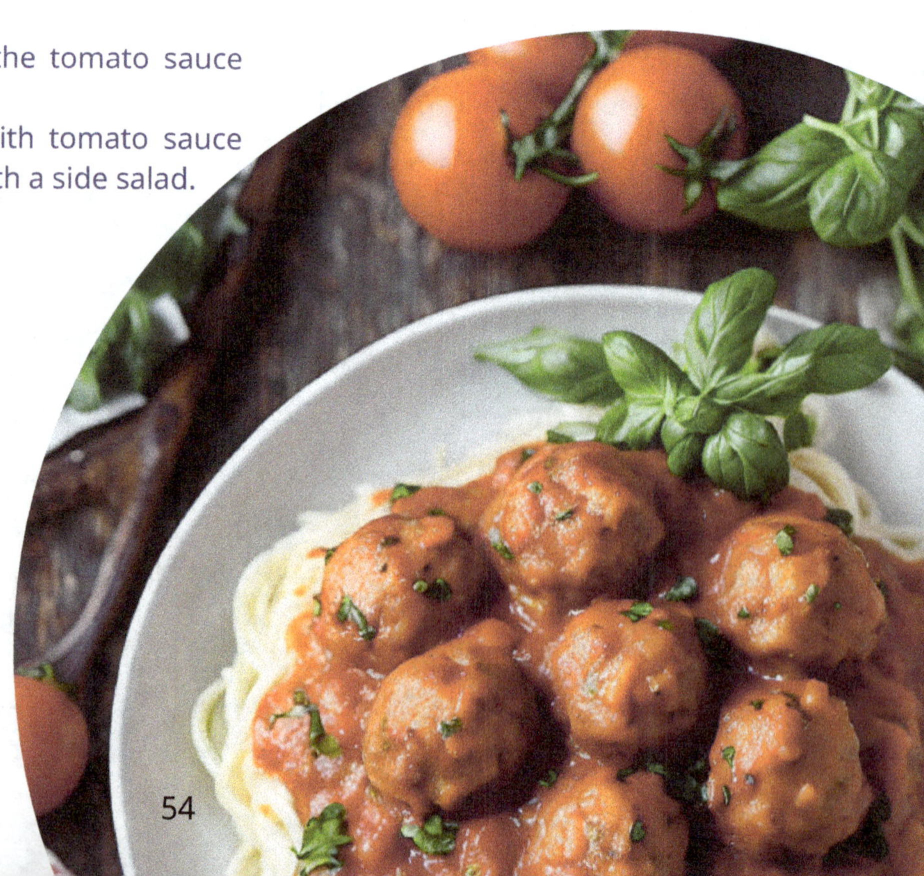

14. Eggplant Parmesan

Preparation Time: 30 minutes
Cook Time: 45 minutes
Total Time: 1 hour 15 minutes

Serves: 4

Ingredients:

 2 medium eggplants, sliced into 1/2-inch thick rounds
- 1 cup all-purpose flour
- 2 eggs, beaten
- 1 cup breadcrumbs
- 1/2 cup grated Parmesan cheese
- 2 tablespoons olive oil
- 1 (24 oz) jar marinara sauce
- 2 cups shredded mozzarella cheese
- Fresh basil, for garnish

Directions:

1. Preheat the oven to 375°F.
2. Set up three shallow dishes: one with the flour, one with the beaten eggs, and one with the breadcrumbs and Parmesan cheese mixed together.
3. Dredge the eggplant slices in the flour, then dip them in the egg, and finally coat them in the breadcrumb mixture.
4. Heat the olive oil in a large skillet over medium heat. Working in batches, fry the breaded eggplant slices for 2-3 minutes per side, or until golden brown. Transfer the fried eggplant to a paper towel-lined plate.
5. Spread 1/2 cup of the marinara sauce in the bottom of a 9x13-inch baking dish.
6. Arrange a layer of the fried eggplant slices in the baking dish. Top with 1/2 cup of the marinara sauce and 1/2 cup of the mozzarella cheese.
7. Repeat the layers of eggplant, sauce, and mozzarella until all the ingredients are used up, ending with the mozzarella cheese.
8. Bake the eggplant parmesan for 30-35 minutes, or until the cheese is melted and bubbly.
9. Let the eggplant parmesan cool for 5-10 minutes before serving. Garnish with fresh basil.

Nutrition Facts (per serving):
- Calories: 450
- Total Fat: 20g
- Saturated Fat: 8g
- Cholesterol: 105mg
- Sodium: 1,050mg
- Total Carbohydrates: 48g
- Dietary Fiber: 8g
- Sugars: 10g
- Protein: 22g

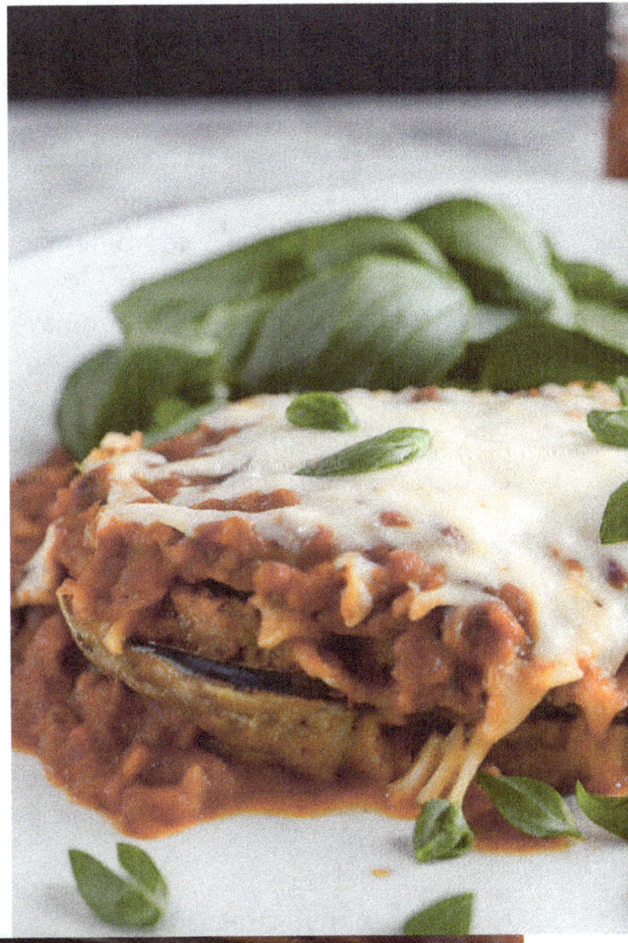

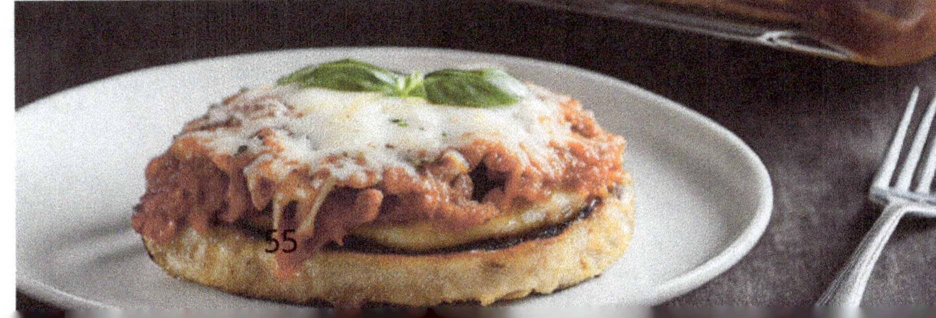

15. Grilled Portobello Mushrooms with Quinoa

Preparation Time: 20 minutes
Cook Time: 20 minutes
Total Time: 40 minutes

Serves: 4

Directions:

1. Preheat grill to medium-high heat.

2. In a small bowl, whisk together the olive oil, balsamic vinegar, salt, and black pepper.

3. Brush the portobello mushrooms with the oil mixture, making sure to coat both sides.

4. Grill the mushrooms for 5-7 minutes per side, or until they are tender and slightly charred.

5. Remove the mushrooms from the grill and let them cool slightly.

6. In a medium bowl, combine the cooked quinoa, diced tomatoes, crumbled feta cheese, chopped basil, and lemon juice. Stir to mix well.

7. Place the grilled portobello mushrooms on a serving plate and spoon the quinoa mixture into the center of each mushroom.

8. Serve the stuffed portobello mushrooms immediately.

Nutrition Facts (per serving):
- Calories: 220
- Total Fat: 12g
- Saturated Fat: 3g
- Cholesterol: 15mg
- Sodium: 480mg
- Total Carbohydrates: 20g
- Dietary Fiber: 4g
- Sugars: 3g
- Protein: 10g

Ingredients:

4 large portobello mushrooms, stems removed
- 2 tablespoons olive oil
- 1 teaspoon balsamic vinegar
- 1/2 teaspoon salt
- 1/4 teaspoon black pepper
- 1 cup cooked quinoa
- 1/2 cup diced tomatoes
- 1/4 cup crumbled feta cheese
- 2 tablespoons chopped fresh basil
- 1 tablespoon lemon juice

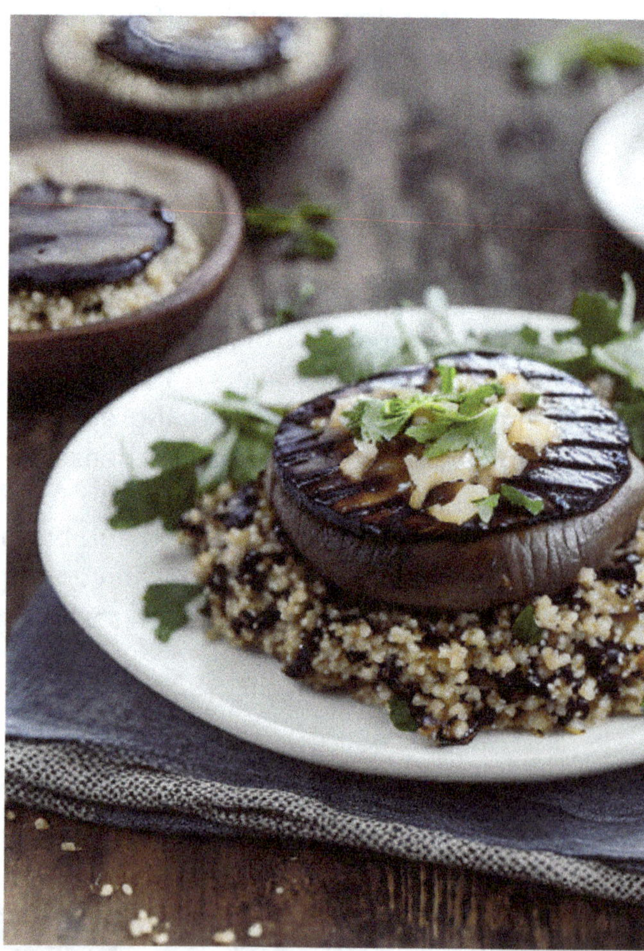

16. Cabbage Rolls with Ground Beef and Rice

Preparation Time: 30 minutes
Cook Time: 1 hour 30 minutes
Total Time: 2 hours

Serves: 6

Directions:

1. Bring a large pot of water to a boil. Core the cabbage and carefully place it in the boiling water. Cook for 3-5 minutes, until the outer leaves are softened. Remove the cabbage from the water and let it cool.
2. Carefully peel off the softened cabbage leaves, keeping them intact. You should have about 12-14 leaves.
3. In a large bowl, combine the ground beef, cooked rice, onion, garlic, oregano, salt, and black pepper. Mix well.
4. Place about 1/4 cup of the beef and rice mixture onto the center of each cabbage leaf. Fold the sides of the leaf over the filling, then roll up tightly.
5. Arrange the stuffed cabbage rolls in a large baking dish.
6. In a medium bowl, mix together the crushed tomatoes, tomato sauce, brown sugar, and Worcestershire sauce. Pour the sauce over the cabbage rolls.
7. Cover the baking dish with foil and bake at 350°F for 1 hour and 15 minutes, or until the cabbage rolls are tender and the filling is cooked through.
8. Serve the cabbage rolls warm, with the tomato sauce spooned over the top.

Nutrition Facts (per serving):
- Calories: 300
- Total Fat: 12g
- Saturated Fat: 4.5g
- Cholesterol: 55mg
- Sodium: 750mg
- Total Carbohydrates: 30g
- Dietary Fiber: 5g
- Sugars: 12g
- Protein: 20g

Ingredients:

 1 large head green cabbage
- 1 pound ground beef
- 1 cup cooked white rice
- 1 onion, finely chopped
- 2 cloves garlic, minced
- 1 teaspoon dried oregano
- 1/2 teaspoon salt
- 1/4 teaspoon black pepper
- 1 (28 oz) can crushed tomatoes
- 1 (8 oz) can tomato sauce
- 1 tablespoon brown sugar
- 1 teaspoon Worcestershire sauce

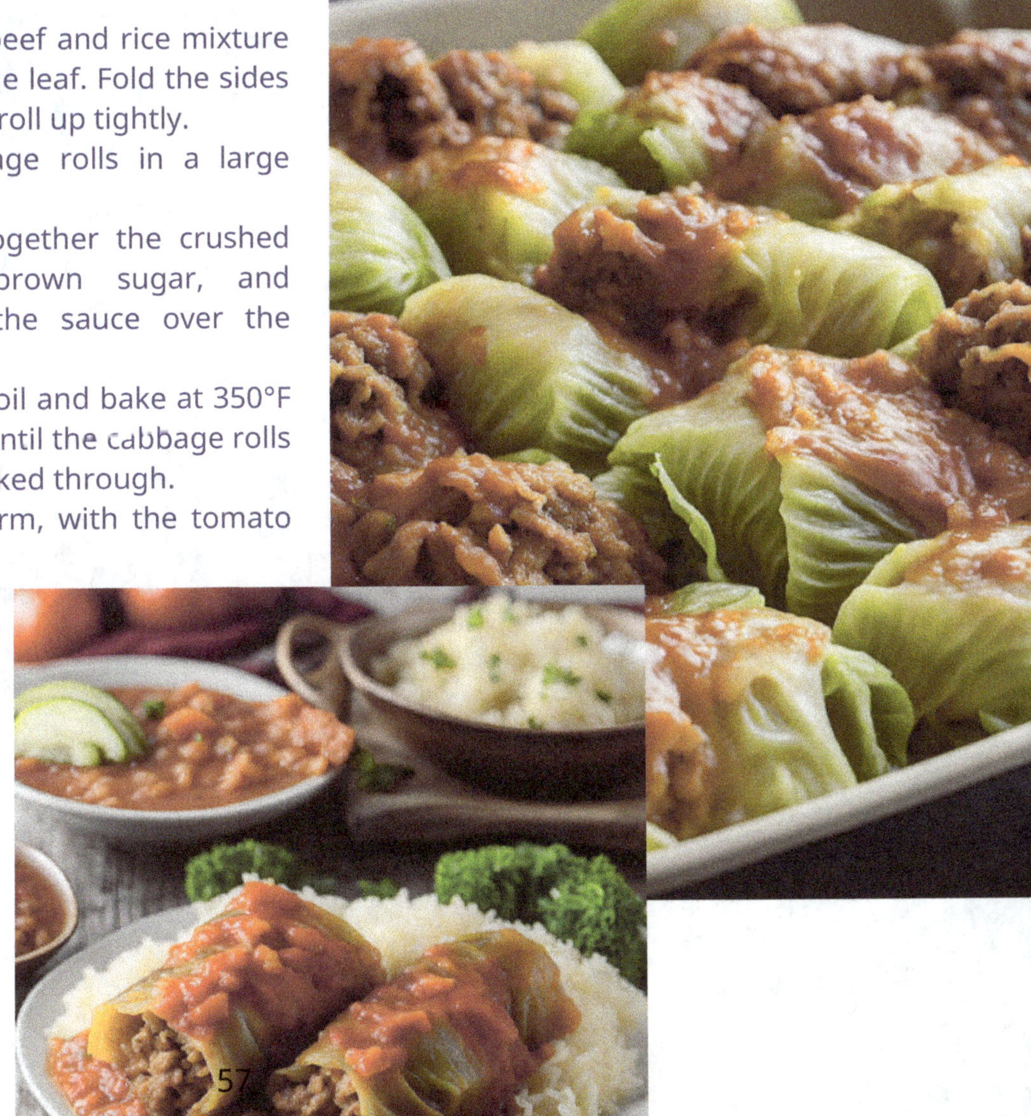

1. Carrot and Celery Sticks with Hummus

Preparation Time: 10 minutes
Total Time: 10 minutes

Serves: 2

Ingredients:

2 medium carrots, peeled and cut into sticks
- 2 celery stalks, cut into sticks
- 1/2 cup hummus

Directions:

1. Arrange the carrot and celery sticks on a plate or in a bowl.

2. Serve the hummus alongside the vegetable sticks for dipping.

Nutrition Facts (per serving):
- Calories: 120
- Total Fat: 6g
- Saturated Fat: 1g
- Cholesterol: 0mg
- Sodium: 360mg
- Total Carbohydrates: 14g
- Dietary Fiber: 5g
- Sugars: 5g
- Protein: 4g

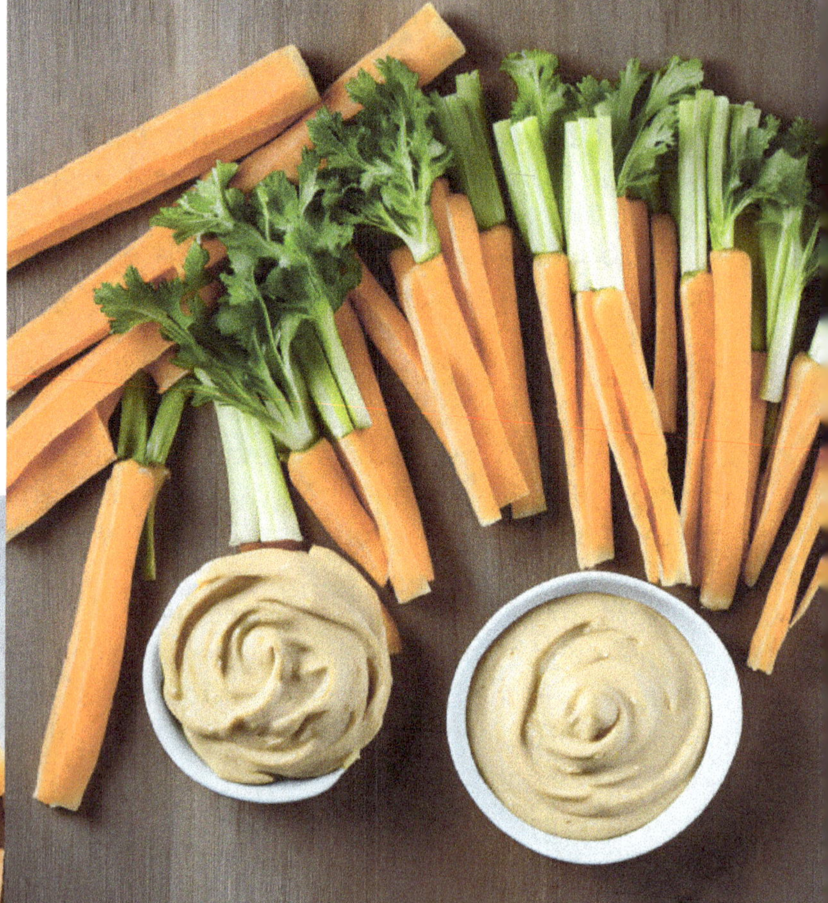

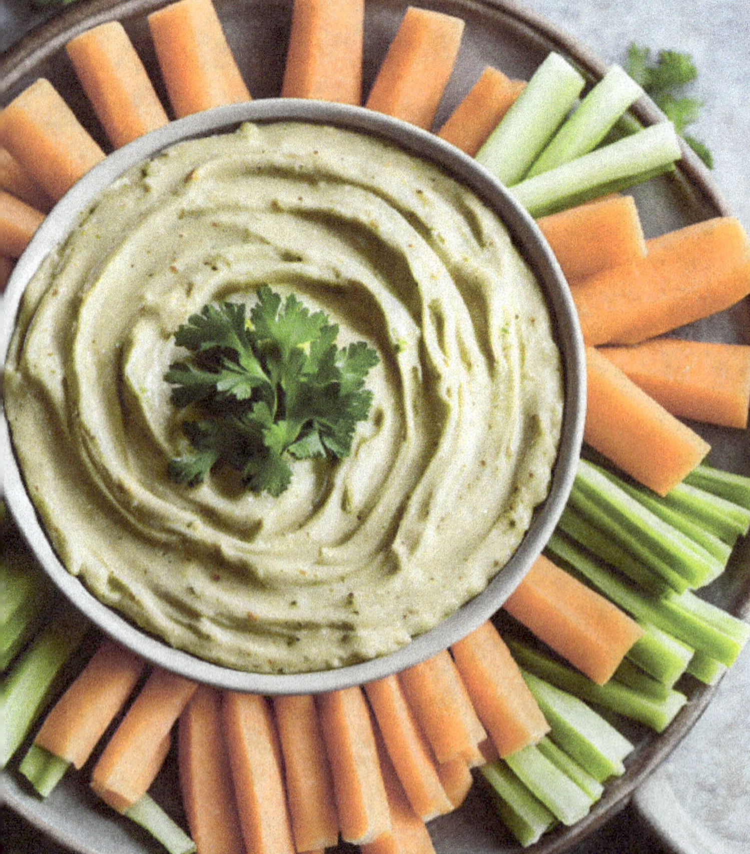

2. Almonds and Dark Chocolate

Preparation Time: 5 minutes
Total Time: 5 minutes

Serves: 1

Ingredients:

 1/4 cup raw almonds
- 1 ounce dark chocolate (70% cacao or higher), chopped

Directions:

1. Combine the almonds and chopped dark chocolate in a small bowl.

2. Enjoy the almonds and dark chocolate as a snack.

Nutrition Facts (per serving):
- Calories: 250
- Total Fat: 19g
- Saturated Fat: 6g
- Cholesterol: 0mg
- Sodium: 0mg
- Total Carbohydrates: 16g
- Dietary Fiber: 6g
- Sugars: 8g
- Protein: 7g

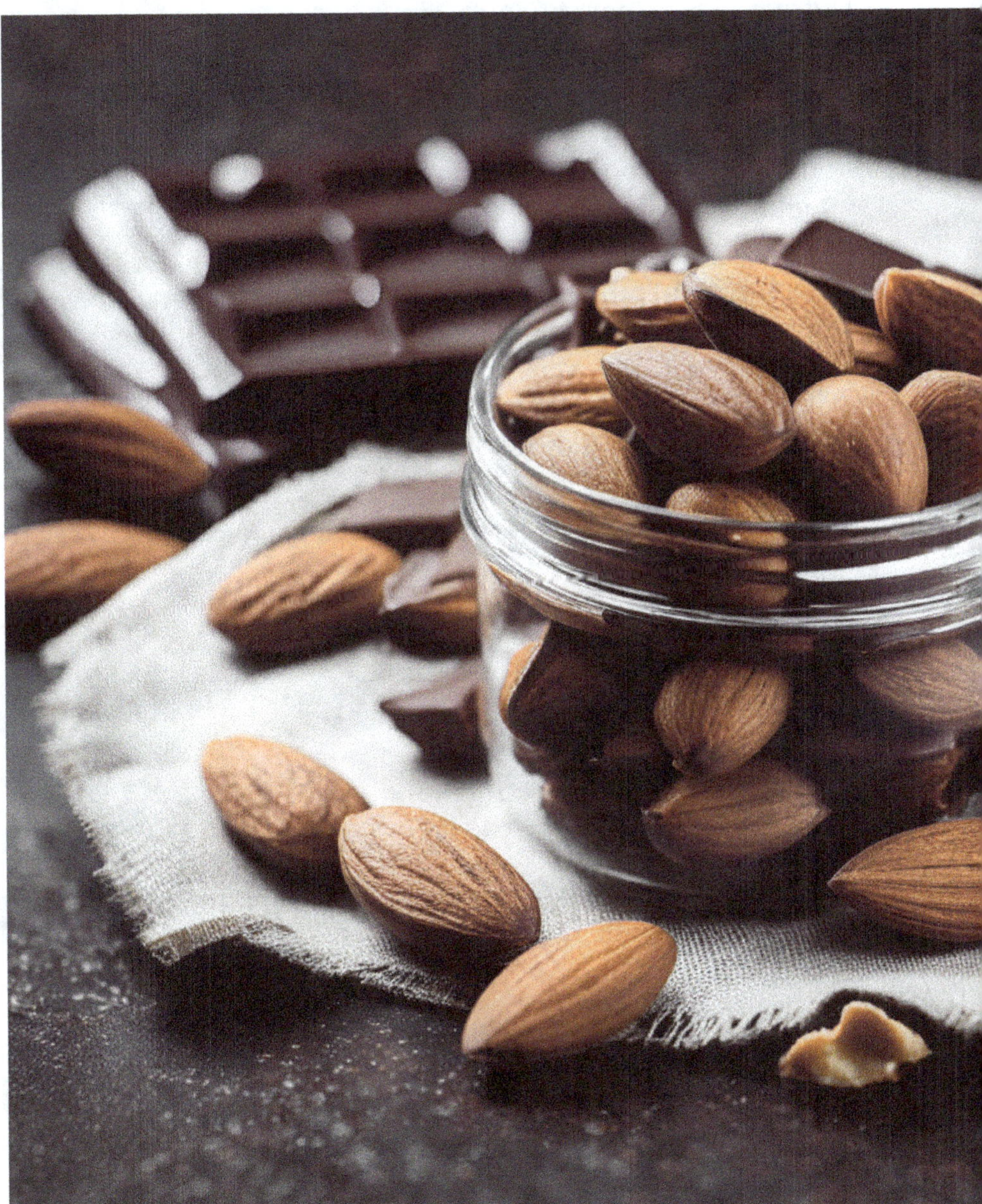

3. Apple Slices with Peanut Butter

Preparation Time: 5 minutes
Total Time: 5 minutes

Serves: 1

Ingredients:

 1 medium apple, cored and sliced
- 2 tablespoons natural peanut butter

Directions:

1. Arrange the apple slices on a plate or in a bowl.

2. Serve the peanut butter alongside the apple slices for dipping.

Nutrition Facts (per serving):
- Calories: 210
- Total Fat: 12g
- Saturated Fat: 2g
- Cholesterol: 0mg
- Sodium: 105mg
- Total Carbohydrates: 22g
- Dietary Fiber: 5g
- Sugars: 16g
- Protein: 7g

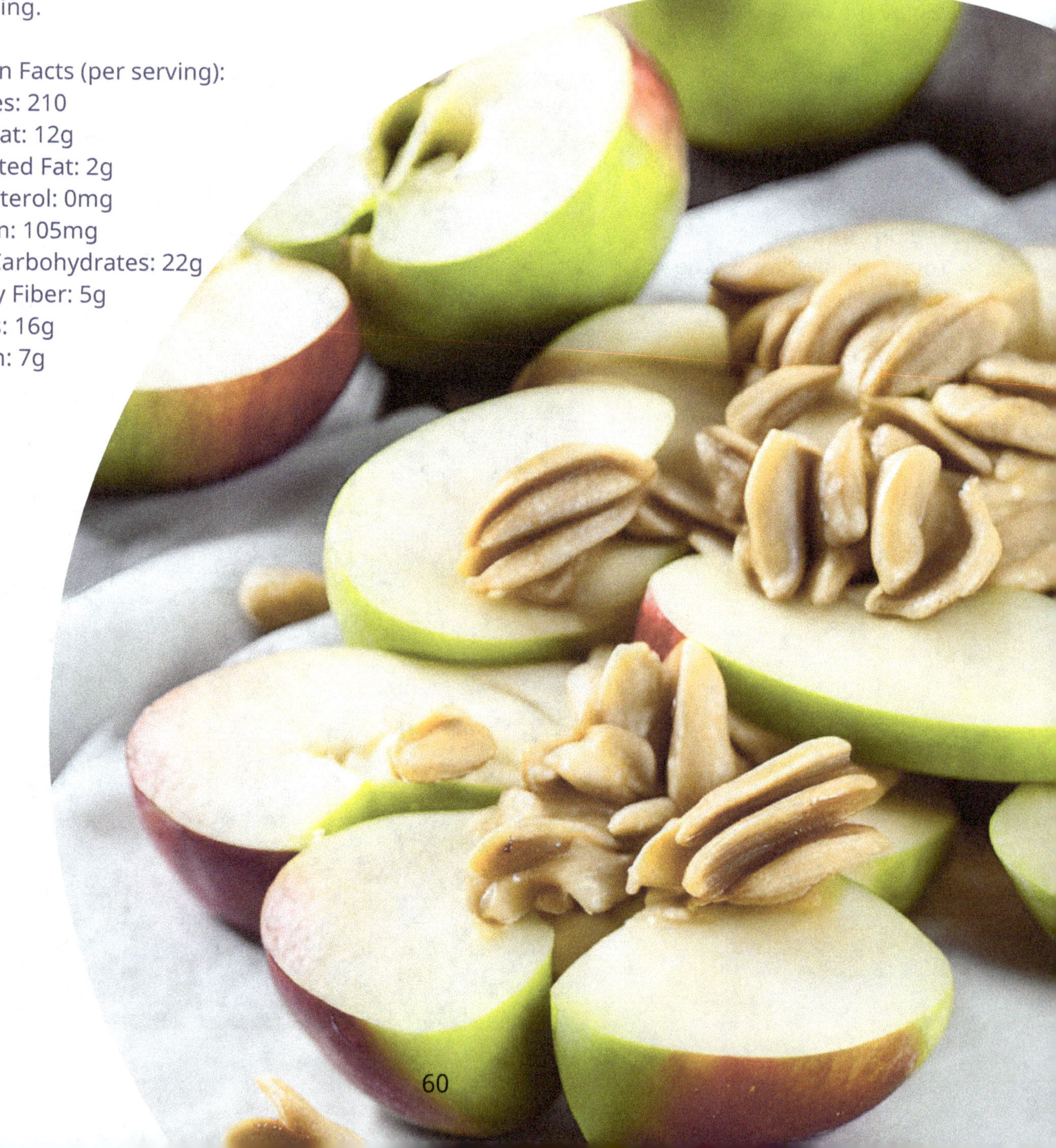

4. Greek Yogurt with Honey and Walnuts

Preparation Time: 5 minutes
Total Time: 5 minutes

Serves: 1

Ingredients:

 1 cup plain Greek yogurt
- 1 tablespoon honey
- 2 tablespoons chopped walnuts

Directions:

1. Place the Greek yogurt in a bowl.

2. Drizzle the honey over the yogurt.

3. Sprinkle the chopped walnuts on top.

Nutrition Facts (per serving):
- Calories: 220
- Total Fat: 12g
- Saturated Fat: 2g
- Cholesterol: 15mg
- Sodium: 55mg
- Total Carbohydrates: 16g
- Dietary Fiber: 2g
- Sugars: 13g
- Protein: 15g

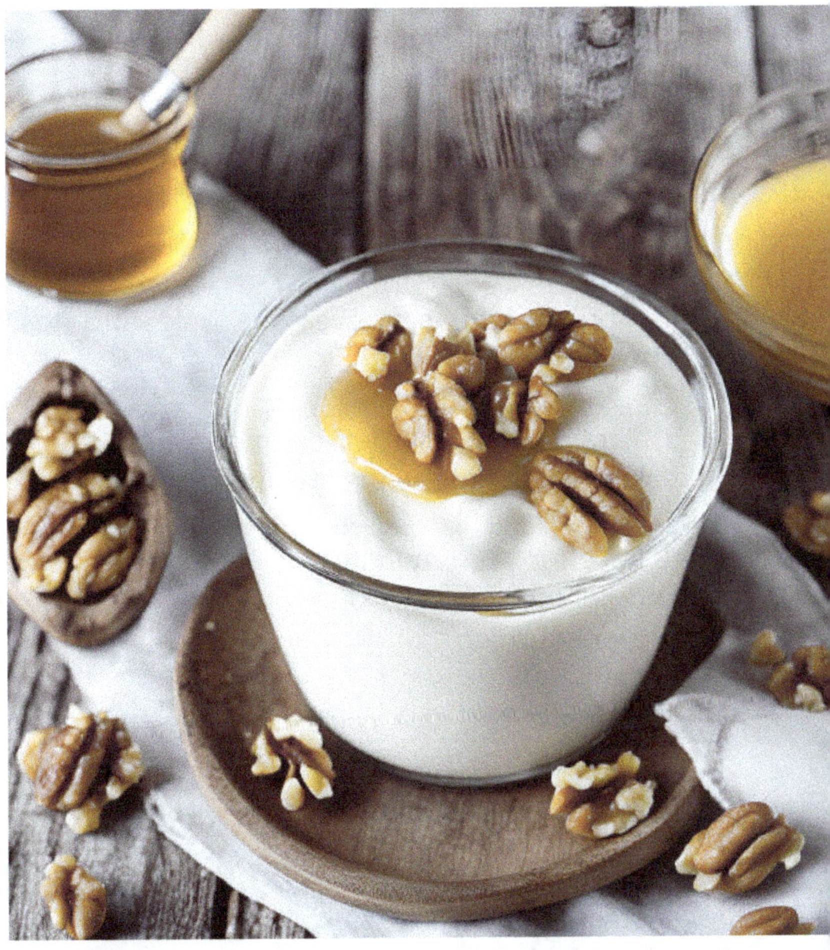

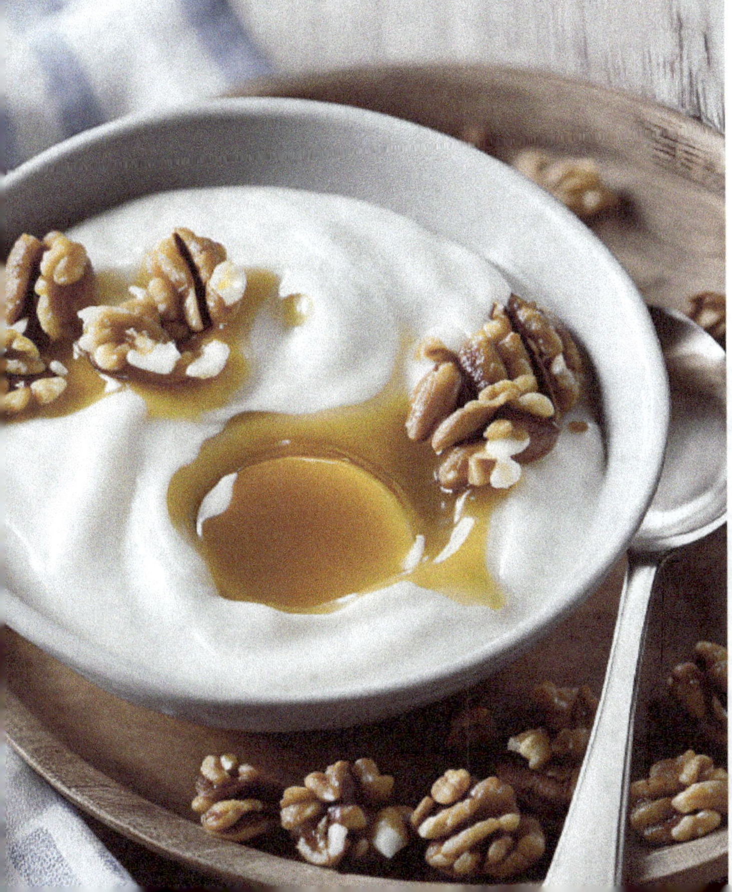

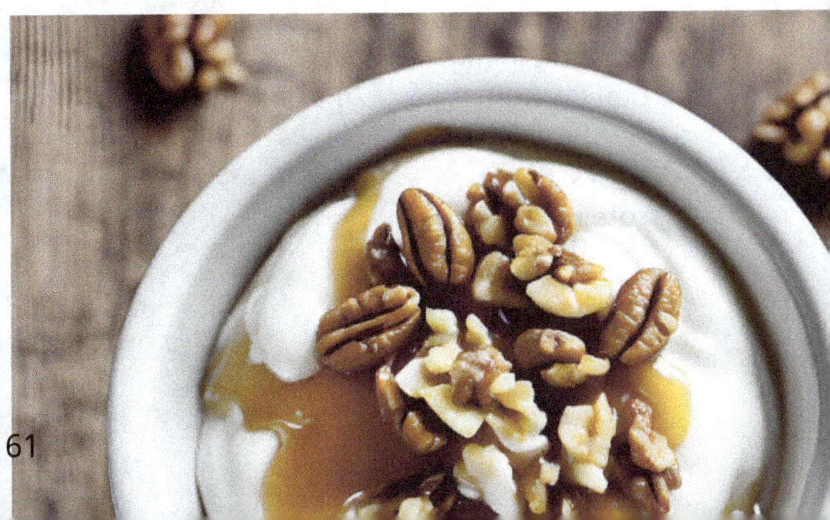

5. Kale Chips

Preparation Time: 10 minutes
Cook Time: 12-15 minutes
Total Time: 22-25 minutes

Serves: 2

Directions:

1. Preheat the oven to 350°F.

2. Wash and thoroughly dry the kale leaves. Place them in a large bowl.

3. Drizzle the olive oil over the kale and use your hands to massage the oil into the leaves, making sure they are all evenly coated.

4. Sprinkle the salt over the kale and toss to distribute.

5. Arrange the kale leaves in a single layer on a baking sheet lined with parchment paper.

6. Bake for 12-15 minutes, or until the kale is crispy and lightly browned. Keep a close eye on them to prevent burning.

7. Remove the kale chips from the oven and let them cool for a few minutes before serving.

Nutrition Facts (per serving):
- Calories: 80
- Total Fat: 5g
- Saturated Fat: 1g
- Cholesterol: 0mg
- Sodium: 230mg
- Total Carbohydrates: 7g
- Dietary Fiber: 2g
- Sugars: 0g
- Protein: 3g

Ingredients:
 1 bunch kale, stems removed and leaves torn into bite-sized pieces
- 1 tablespoon olive oil
- 1/4 teaspoon salt

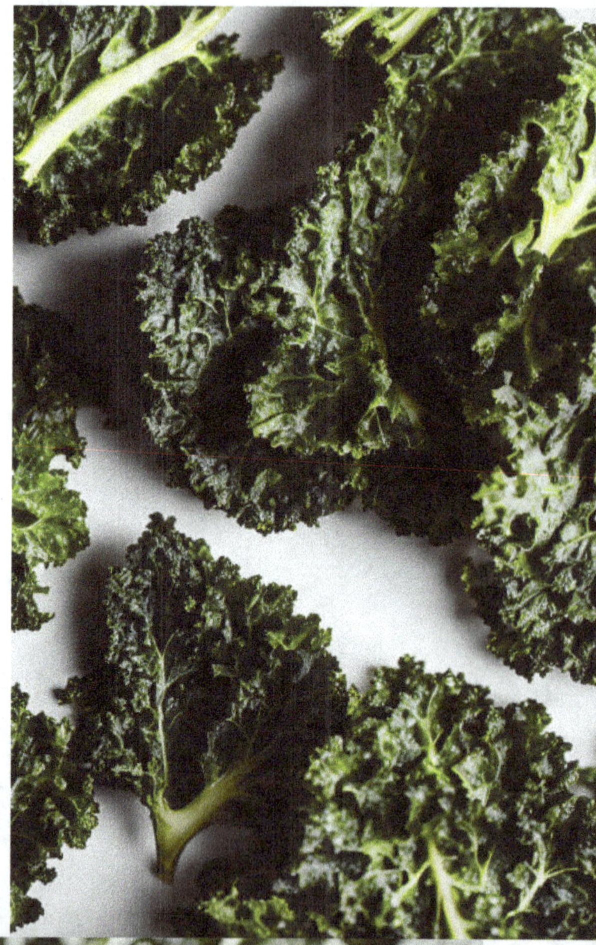

6. Edamame with Sea Salt

Preparation Time: 5 minutes
Cook Time: 5 minutes
Total Time: 10 minutes

Serves: 2

Directions:

1. Bring a medium pot of water to a boil.
2. Add the frozen edamame and cook for 5 minutes, or until tender.
3. Drain the edamame and transfer to a serving bowl.
4. Sprinkle the sea salt over the edamame and toss to coat.
5. Serve the edamame warm, with the pods intact.

Nutrition Facts (per serving):
- Calories: 100
- Total Fat: 5g
- Saturated Fat: 0.5g
- Cholesterol: 0mg
- Sodium: 135mg
- Total Carbohydrates: 9g
- Dietary Fiber: 4g
- Sugars: 2g
- Protein: 8g

Ingredients:

 1 cup frozen edamame, in the pod
- 1/4 teaspoon sea salt

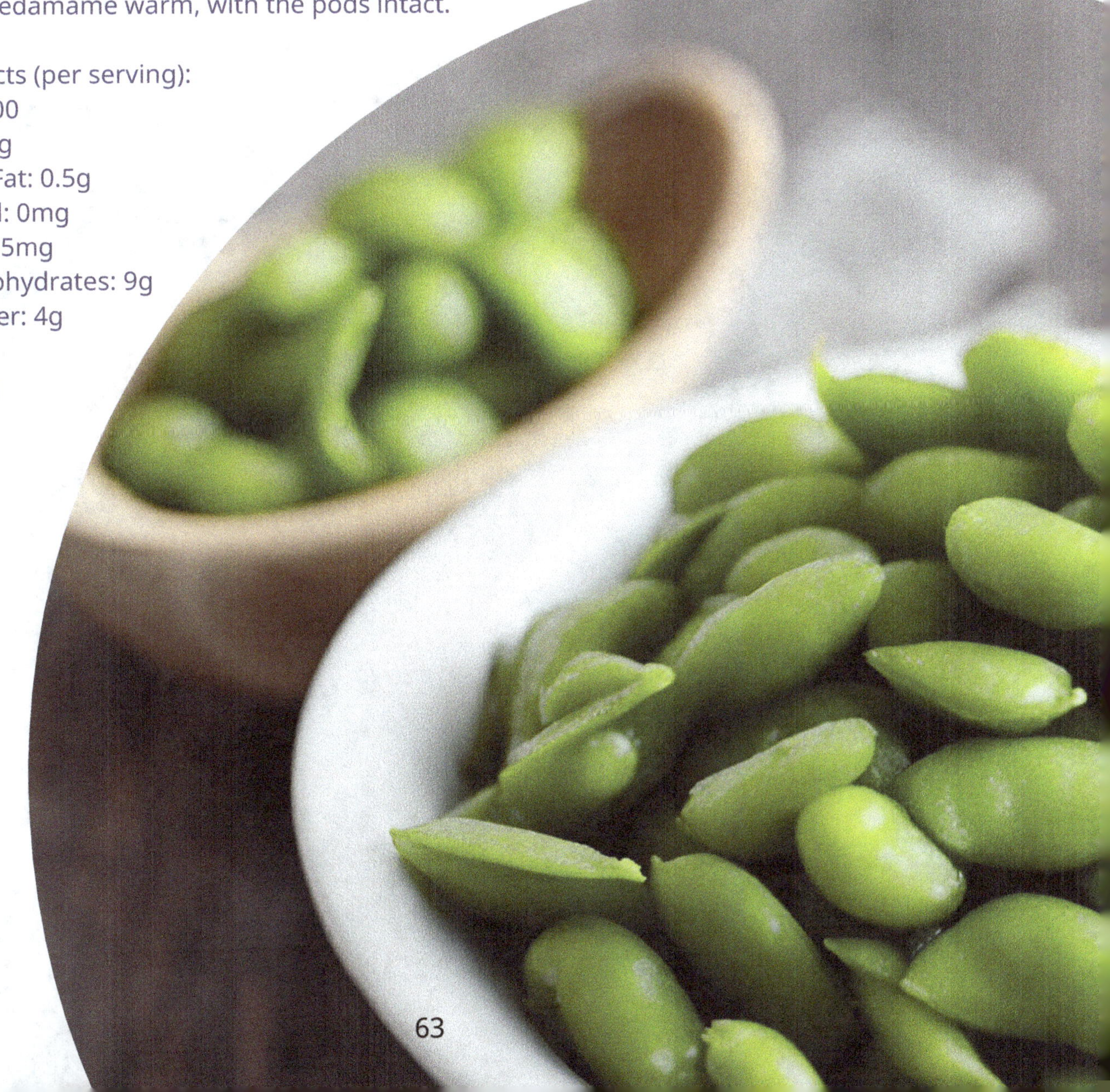

1

7. Homemade Trail Mix with Nuts and Dried Fruit

Preparation Time: 10 minutes
Cook Time: 0 minutes
Total Time: 10 minutes
Serves: 8

Ingredients:

 1 cup raw almonds
- 1 cup raw cashews
- 1 cup raw walnuts
- 1 cup dried cranberries
- 1 cup dried apricots, chopped
- 1/2 cup dark chocolate chips

Directions:

1. In a large bowl, combine all the ingredients and mix well.
2. Transfer the trail mix to an airtight container and store at room temperature for up to 2 weeks.

NUTRITION FACTS (per serving):
Calories: 260
Total Fat: 17g
Saturated Fat: 3g
Cholesterol: 0mg
Sodium: 10mg
Total Carbohydrates: 24g
Dietary Fiber: 4g
Total Sugars: 16g
Protein: 6g

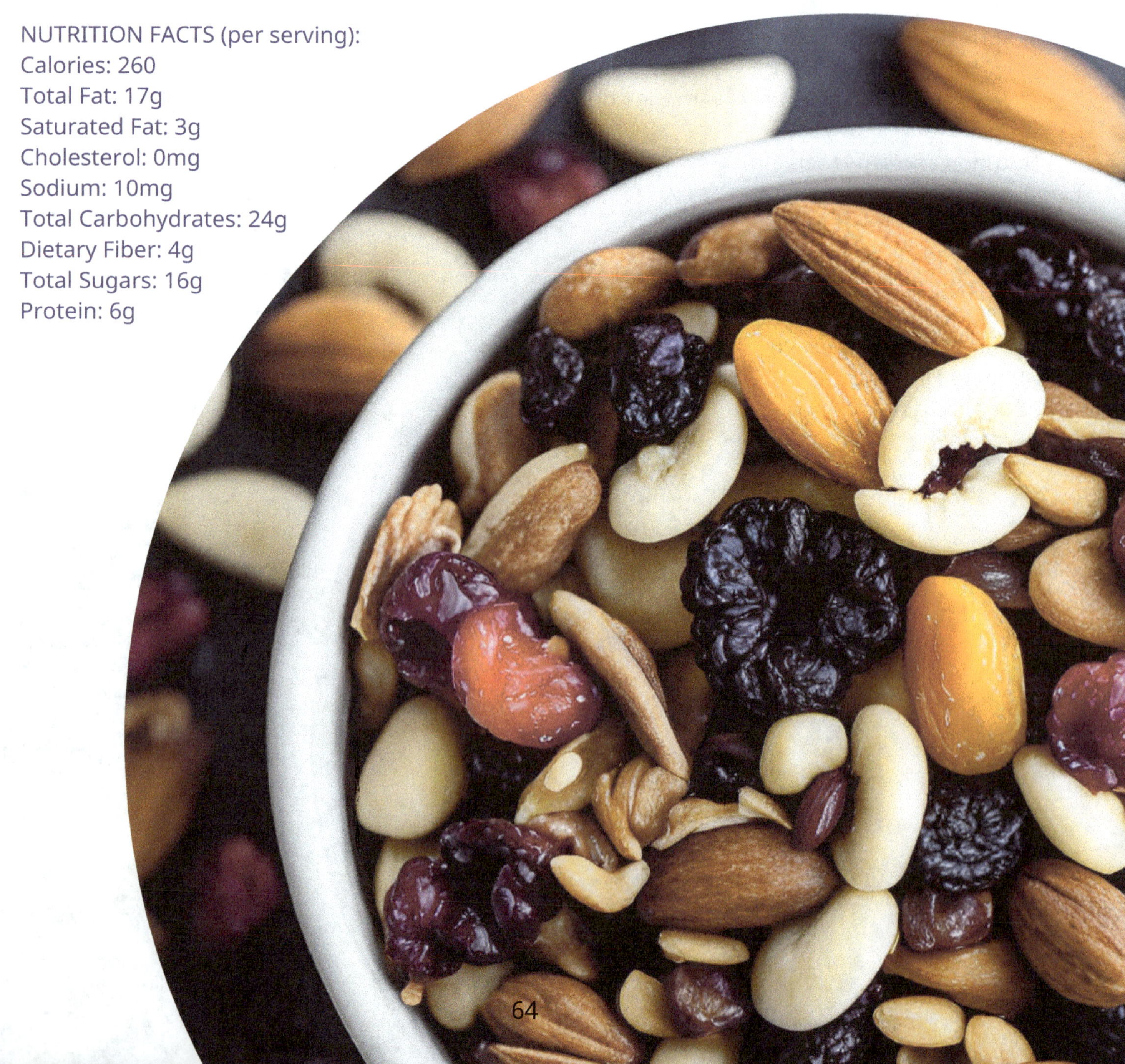

8. Cottage Cheese with Pineapple

Preparation Time: 5 minutes
Cook Time: 0 minutes
Total Time: 5 minutes
Serves: 1

Ingredients:

1/2 cup low-fat cottage cheese
- 1/2 cup diced pineapple

Directions:

1. In a small bowl, combine the cottage cheese and diced pineapple.

2. Serve immediately.

NUTRITION FACTS (per serving):
Calories: 120
Total Fat: 2g
Saturated Fat: 1g
Cholesterol: 10mg
Sodium: 360mg
Total Carbohydrates: 12g
Dietary Fiber: 1g
Total Sugars: 10g
Protein: 14g

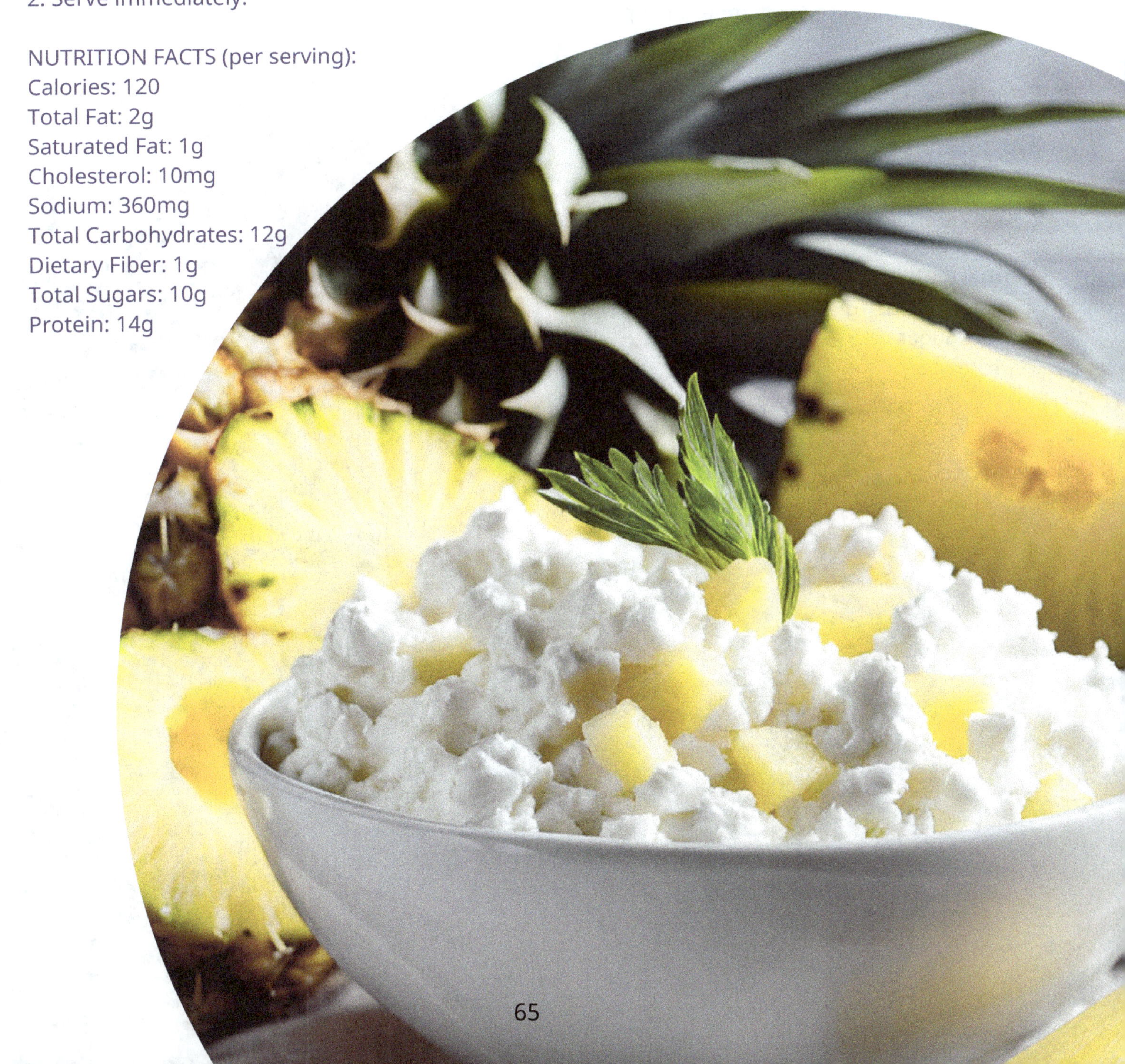

9. Sliced Cucumber with Tzatziki Sauce

Preparation Time: 10 minutes
Cook Time: 0 minutes
Total Time: 10 minutes
Serves: 2

Ingredients:

 1 cucumber, sliced
- 1/2 cup plain Greek yogurt
- 1 tablespoon lemon juice
- 1 garlic clove, minced
- 1 tablespoon chopped fresh dill
- Salt and pepper to taste

Directions:

1. In a small bowl, combine the Greek yogurt, lemon juice, garlic, and dill. Season with salt and pepper to taste.
2. Arrange the sliced cucumber on a plate and serve with the tzatziki sauce on the side.

NUTRITION FACTS (per serving):
Calories: 60
Total Fat: 1g
Saturated Fat: 0g
Cholesterol: 5mg
Sodium: 35mg
Total Carbohydrates: 8g
Dietary Fiber: 1g
Total Sugars: 5g
Protein: 5g

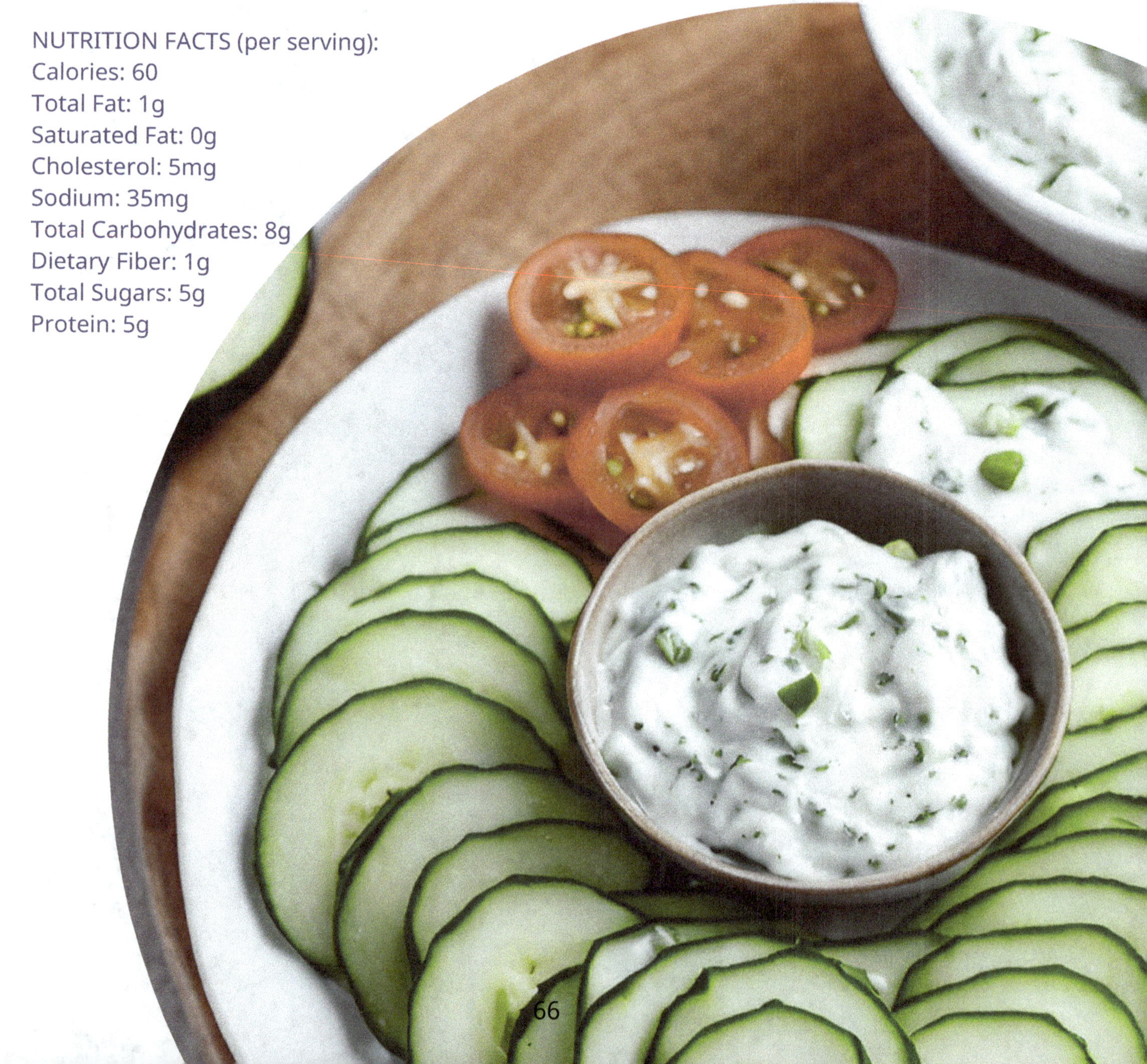

10. Roasted Chickpeas with Spices

Preparation Time: 10 minutes
Cook Time: 25 minutes
Total Time: 35 minutes
Serves: 4

Ingredients:

 1 (15 oz) can chickpeas, drained and rinsed
- 1 tablespoon olive oil
- 1 teaspoon ground cumin
- 1 teaspoon paprika
- 1/2 teaspoon garlic powder
- 1/4 teaspoon cayenne pepper (optional)
- Salt and pepper to taste

Directions:

1. Preheat the oven to 400°F.
2. Pat the chickpeas dry with a paper towel to remove any excess moisture.
3. In a medium bowl, toss the chickpeas with the olive oil, cumin, paprika, garlic powder, and cayenne pepper (if using). Season with salt and pepper.
4. Spread the chickpeas in a single layer on a baking sheet.
5. Roast for 20-25 minutes, stirring halfway, until the chickpeas are crispy.
6. Remove from the oven and let cool slightly before serving.

NUTRITION FACTS (per serving):
Calories: 120
Total Fat: 4g
Saturated Fat: 0.5g
Cholesterol: 0mg
Sodium: 300mg
Total Carbohydrates: 16g
Dietary Fiber: 4g
Total Sugars: 1g
Protein: 5g

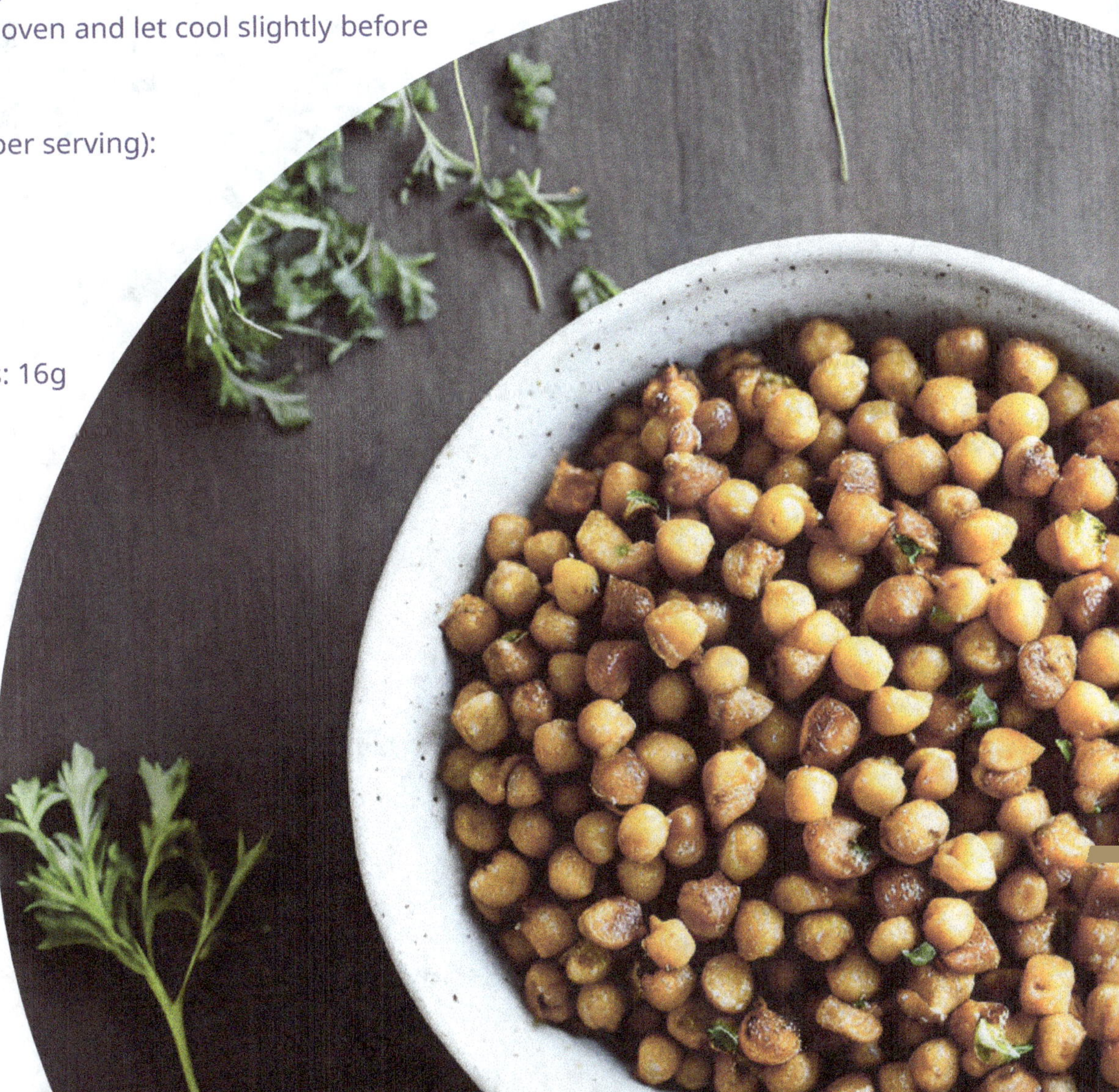

11. Mini Bell Peppers Stuffed with Goat Cheese

Preparation Time: 15 minutes
Cook Time: 15 minutes
Total Time: 30 minutes
Serves: 4

Directions:

1. Preheat the oven to 400°F.

2. In a small bowl, mix together the goat cheese, basil, and lemon juice. Season with salt and pepper.

3. Arrange the bell pepper halves on a baking sheet. Spoon the goat cheese mixture evenly into the pepper halves.

4. Bake for 12-15 minutes, until the peppers are tender and the cheese is lightly browned.
5. Serve warm.

NUTRITION FACTS (per serving):
Calories: 80
Total Fat: 5g
Saturated Fat: 3g
Cholesterol: 10mg
Sodium: 80mg
Total Carbohydrates: 6g
Dietary Fiber: 1g
Total Sugars: 3g
Protein: 4g

Ingredients:

12 mini bell peppers, halved lengthwise and seeds removed
- 4 oz goat cheese, softened
- 2 tablespoons chopped fresh basil
- 1 tablespoon lemon juice
- Salt and pepper to taste

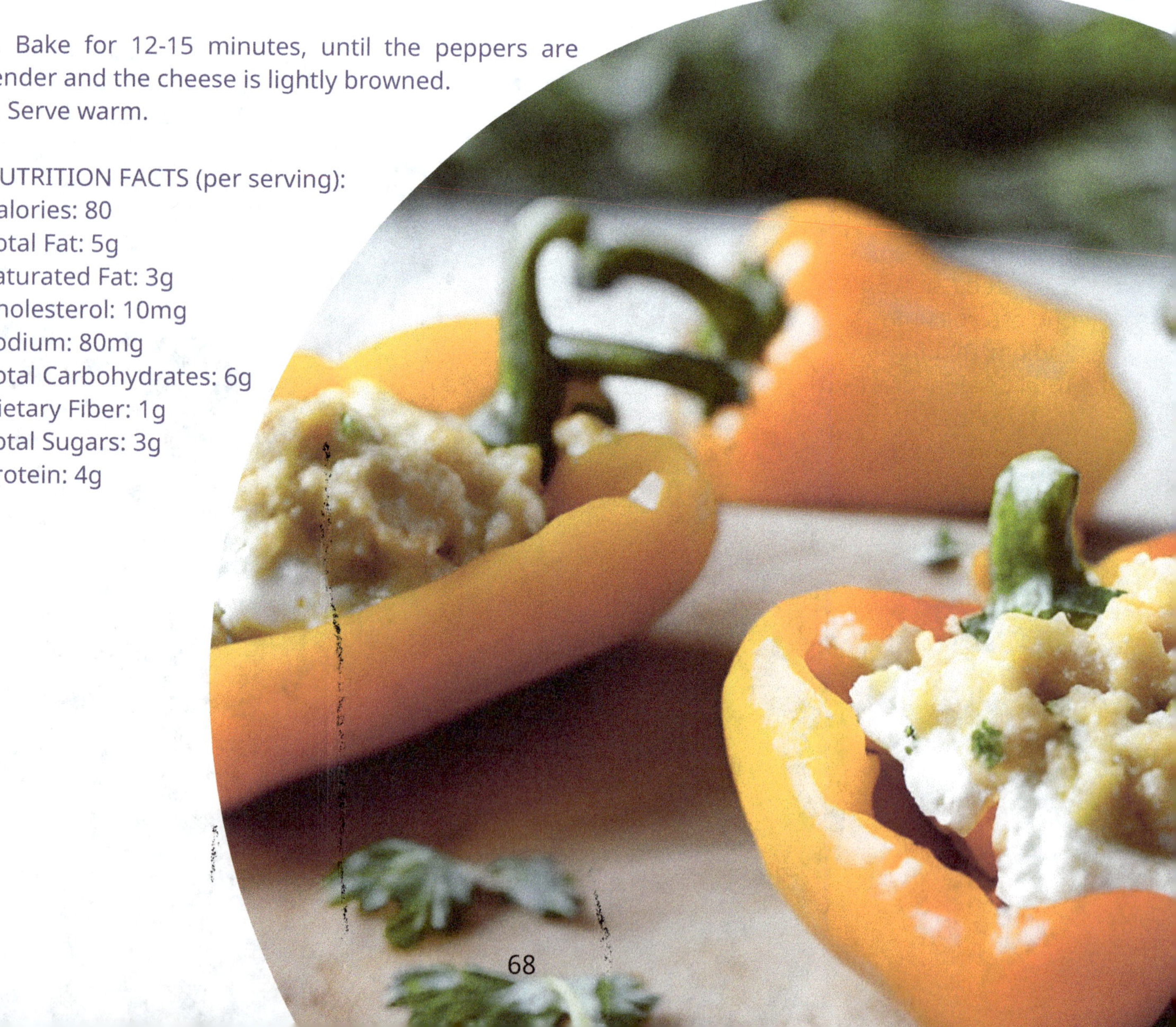

12. Berries and Cottage Cheese

Preparation Time: 5 minutes
Cook Time: 0 minutes
Total Time: 5 minutes
Serves: 1

Ingredients:

 1/2 cup low-fat cottage cheese
- 1/2 cup mixed berries (such as blueberries, raspberries, and/or blackberries)
- 1 teaspoon honey (optional)

Directions:

1. In a small bowl, combine the cottage cheese and mixed berries.

2. If desired, drizzle the honey over the top.

3. Serve immediately.

NUTRITION FACTS (per serving):
Calories: 150
Total Fat: 3g
Saturated Fat: 1g
Cholesterol: 10mg
Sodium: 360mg
Total Carbohydrates: 15g
Dietary Fiber: 3g
Total Sugars: 12g
Protein: 15g

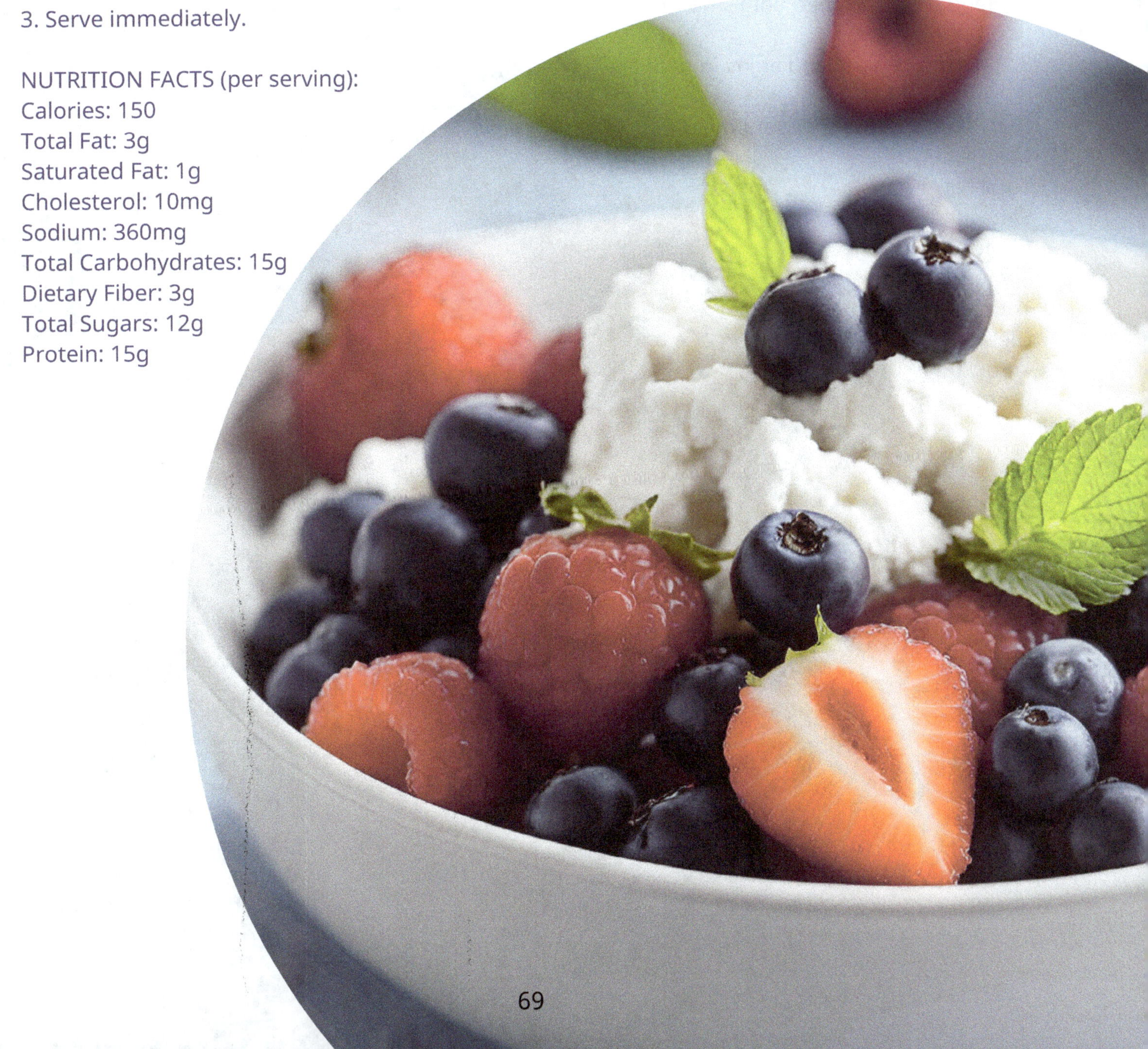

13. Smoothie with Spinach, Banana, and Almond Milk

Preparation Time: 5 minutes
Cook Time: 0 minutes
Total Time: 5 minutes
Serves: 1

Ingredients:

 1 cup unsweetened almond milk
- 1 cup fresh spinach
- 1 ripe banana, frozen
- 1 tablespoon almond butter
- 1 teaspoon honey (optional)

Directions:

1. In a high-speed blender, combine the almond milk, spinach, frozen banana, almond butter, and honey (if using).

2. Blend on high speed until smooth and creamy.

3. Pour into a glass and enjoy immediately.

NUTRITION FACTS (per serving):
Calories: 270
Total Fat: 12g
Saturated Fat: 1g
Cholesterol: 0mg
Sodium: 190mg
Total Carbohydrates: 35g
Dietary Fiber: 7g
Total Sugars: 18g
Protein: 8g

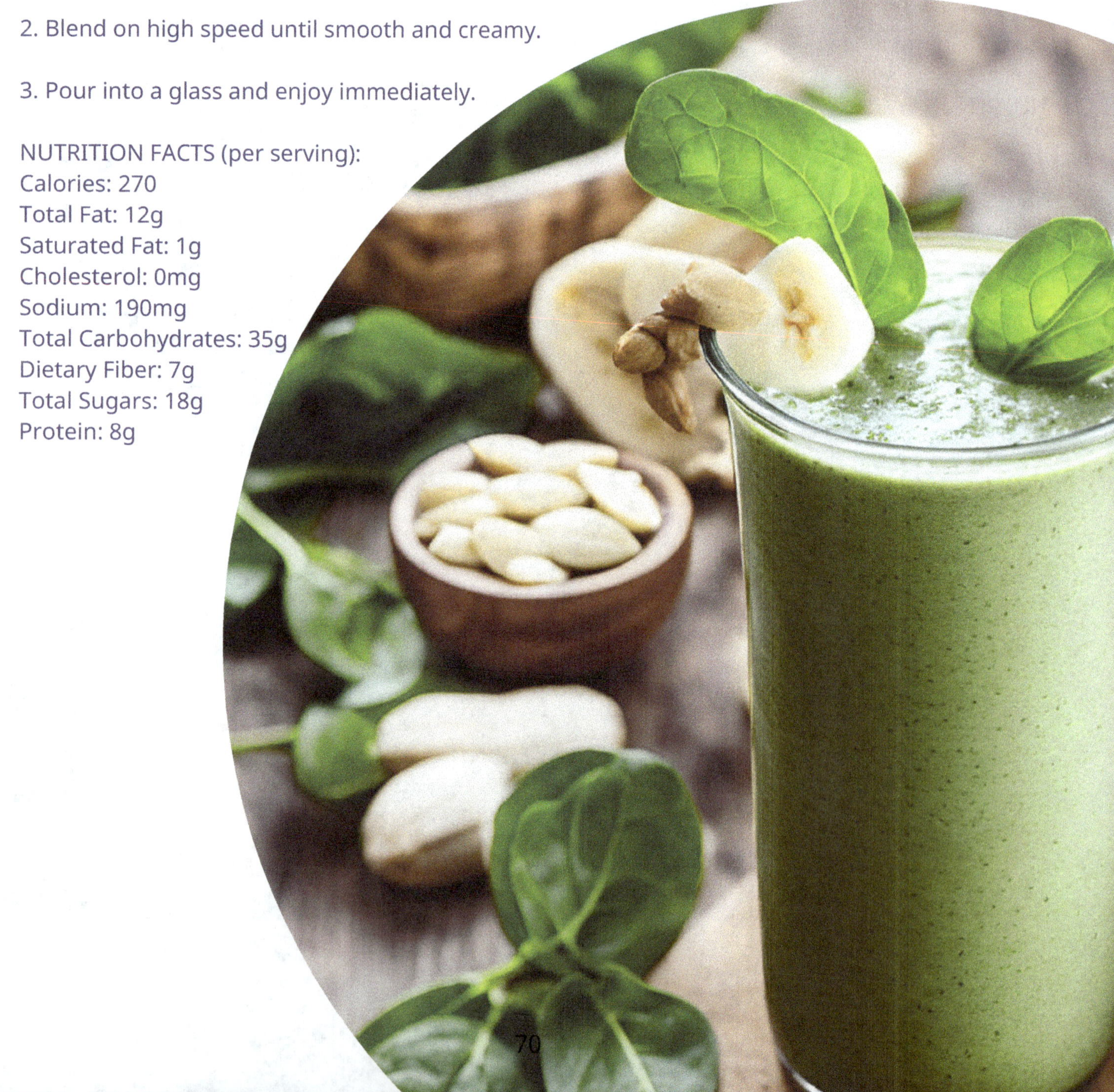

14. Rice Cakes with Avocado

Preparation Time: 5 minutes
Cook Time: 0 minutes
Total Time: 5 minutes
Serves: 1

Ingredients:

 2 whole grain rice cakes
- 1/2 ripe avocado, mashed
- 1 teaspoon lemon juice
- Salt and pepper to taste

Directions:

1. In a small bowl, mash the avocado with the lemon juice. Season with salt and pepper to taste.

2. Spread the mashed avocado evenly over the rice cakes.

3. Serve immediately.

NUTRITION FACTS (per serving):
Calories: 200
Total Fat: 12g
Saturated Fat: 2g
Cholesterol: 0mg
Sodium: 160mg
Total Carbohydrates: 20g
Dietary Fiber: 5g
Total Sugars: 1g
Protein: 4g

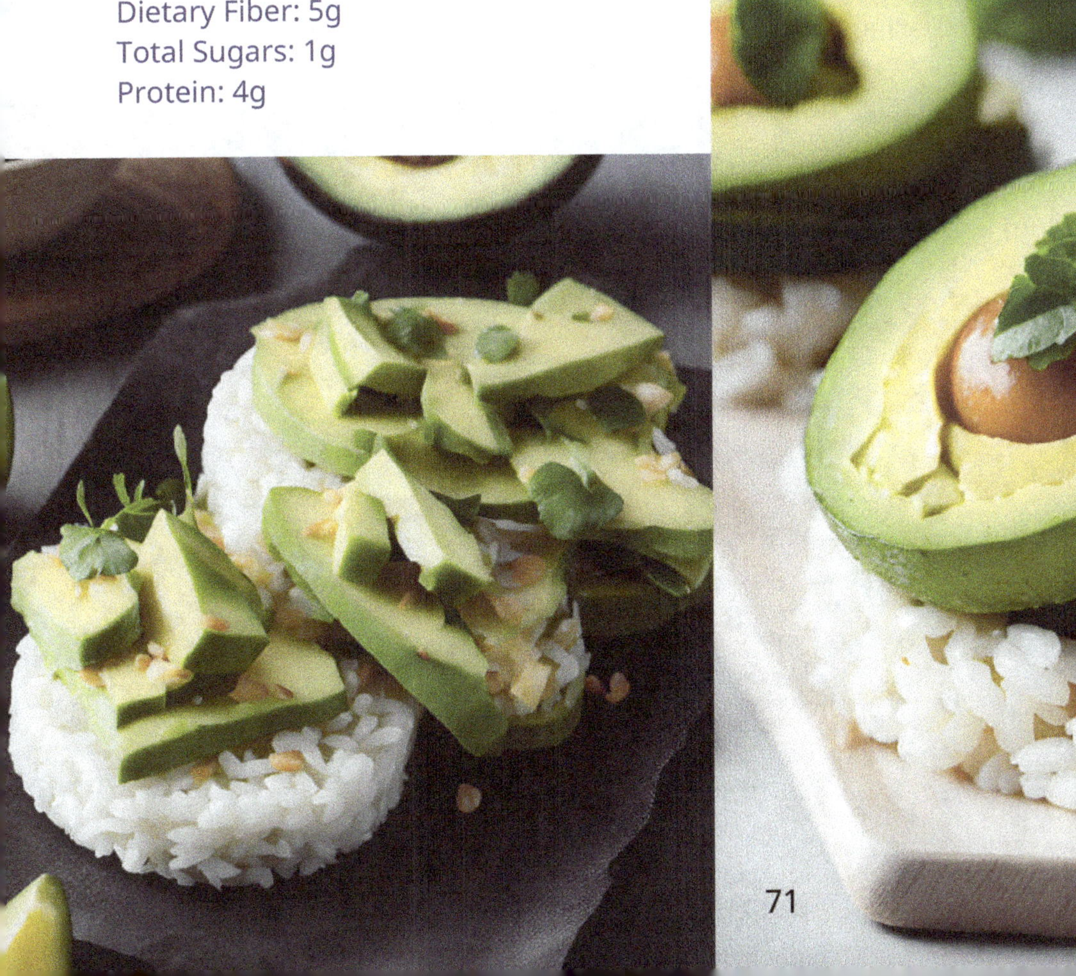

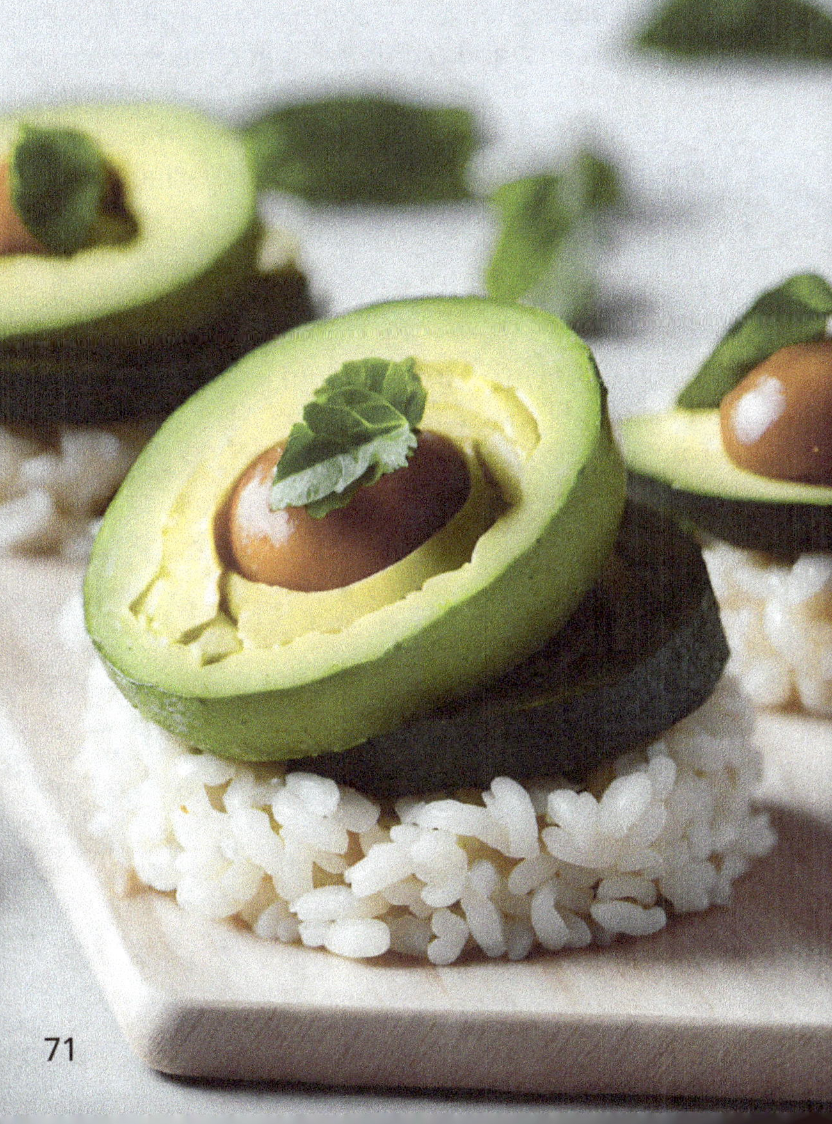

15. Pumpkin Seeds

Preparation Time: 15 minutes
Cook Time: 45 minutes
Total Time: 1 hour
Serves: 4

Directions:

1. Preheat the oven to 400°F.

2. Toss the beet cubes with the olive oil and season with salt and pepper.

3. Spread the beets on a baking sheet and roast for 40-45 minutes, stirring halfway, until tender and caramelized.

4. Allow the beets to cool slightly.

5. In a large salad bowl, combine the roasted beets, mixed greens, and crumbled goat cheese.

6. In a small bowl, whisk together the balsamic vinegar and honey. Drizzle the dressing over the salad and toss to coat.

7. Serve immediately.

NUTRITION FACTS (per serving):
Calories: 190
Total Fat: 12g
Saturated Fat: 4g
Cholesterol: 15mg
Sodium: 310mg
Total Carbohydrates: 16g
Dietary Fiber: 4g
Total Sugars: 10g
Protein: 7g

Ingredients:

4 medium beets, peeled and cut into 1-inch cubes
- 2 tablespoons olive oil
- Salt and pepper to taste
- 4 cups mixed greens
- 4 oz crumbled goat cheese
- 2 tablespoons balsamic vinegar
- 1 tablespoon honey

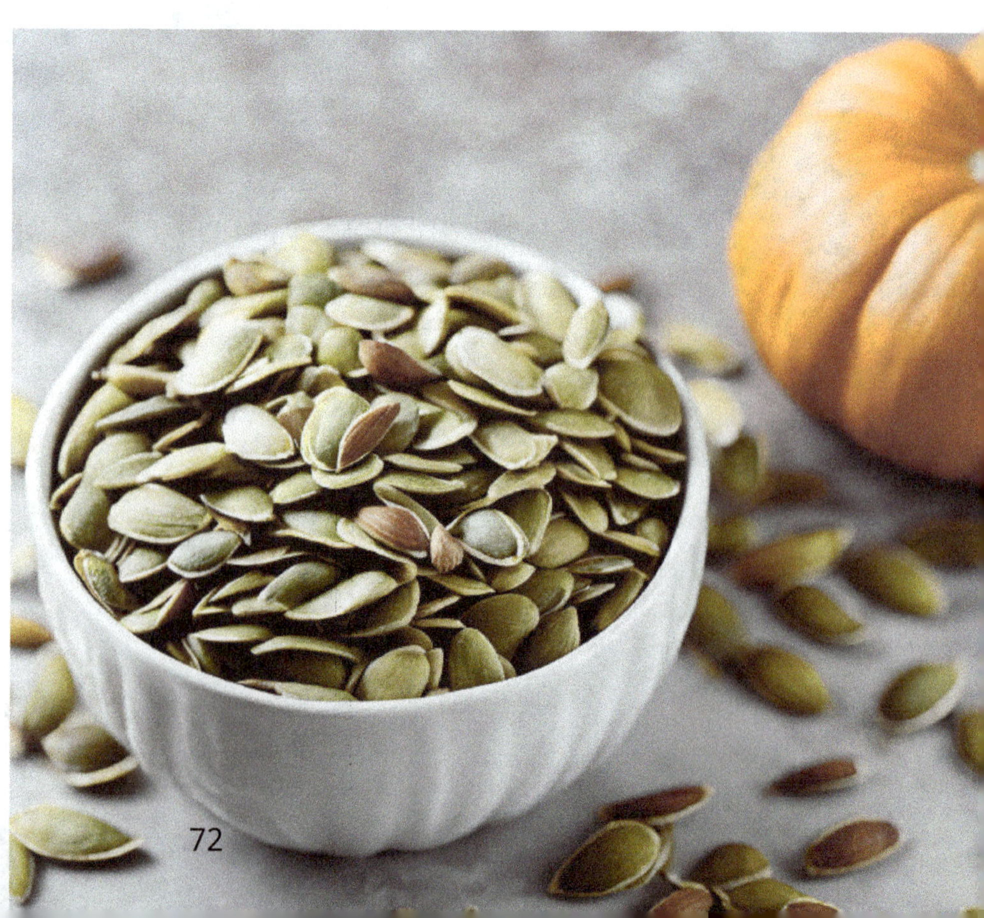

16. Tomato and Mozzarella Skewers

Preparation Time: 10 minutes
Cook Time: 0 minutes
Total Time: 10 minutes
Serves: 4

Ingredients:

 12 cherry tomatoes
- 12 small mozzarella balls (or 1-inch cubes of mozzarella cheese)
- 12 fresh basil leaves
- 2 tablespoons balsamic glaze
- Salt and pepper to taste

Directions:

1. Thread the tomatoes, mozzarella, and basil leaves onto small skewers, alternating the ingredients.

2. Arrange the skewers on a serving platter.

3. Drizzle the balsamic glaze over the skewers and season with salt and pepper.

4. Serve immediately.

NUTRITION FACTS (per serving):
Calories: 80
Total Fat: 5g
Saturated Fat: 3g
Cholesterol: 15mg
Sodium: 220mg
Total Carbohydrates: 4g
Dietary Fiber: 1g
Total Sugars: 3g
Protein: 6g

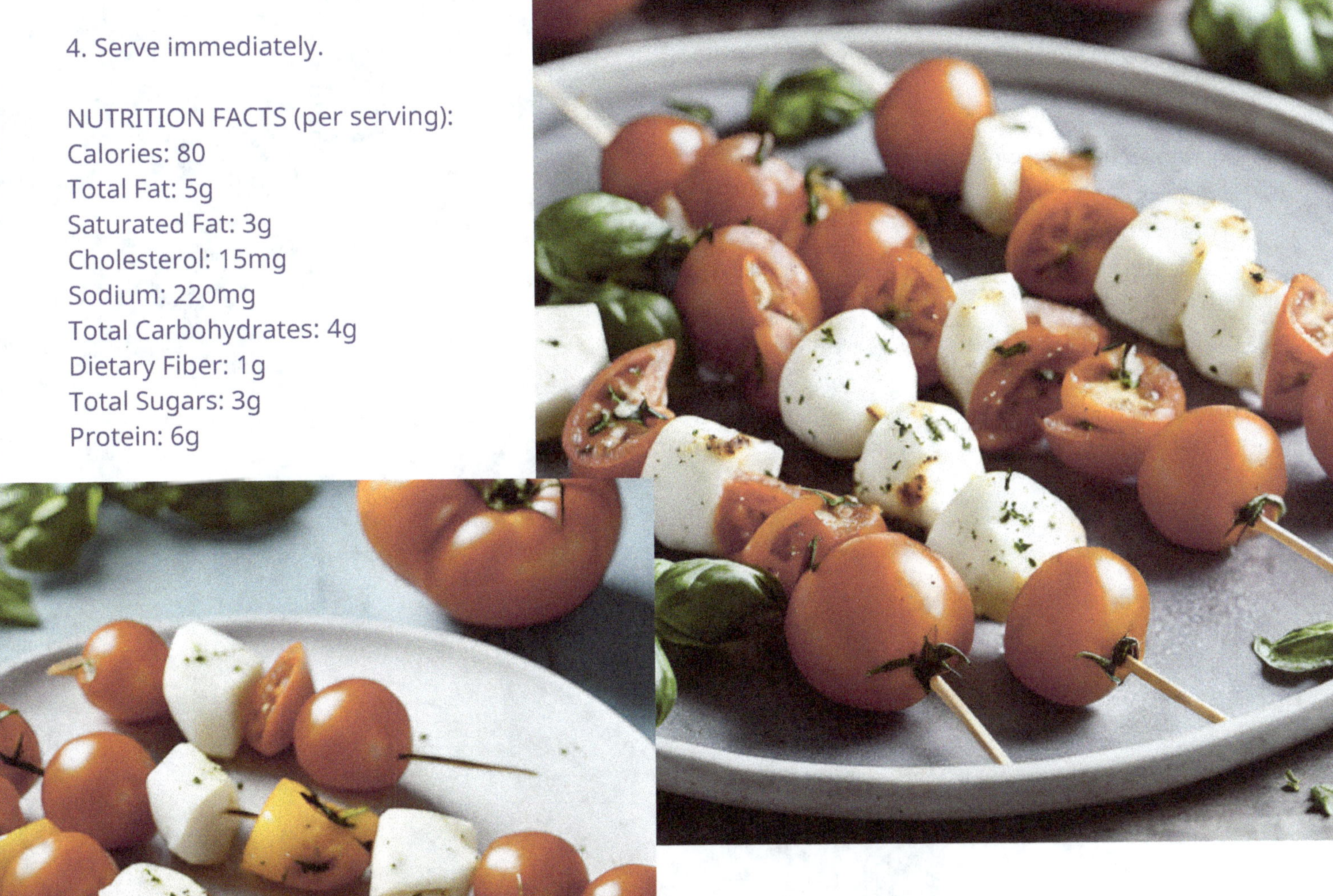

1. Chia Seed Pudding with Mango

Preparation Time: 10 minutes
Chilling Time: 4 hours
Total Time: 4 hours 10 minutes
Serves: 2

Ingredients:

 1/4 cup chia seeds
- 1 cup unsweetened almond milk
- 1 tablespoon honey
- 1/2 teaspoon vanilla extract
- 1 cup diced mango

Directions:

1. In a medium bowl, whisk together the chia seeds, almond milk, honey, and vanilla extract.

2. Cover and refrigerate for at least 4 hours, or overnight, stirring occasionally, until thickened.

3. Divide the chia seed pudding between two serving bowls or glasses.

4. Top each serving with 1/2 cup of diced mango.
5. Serve chilled.

NUTRITION FACTS (per serving):
Calories: 210
Total Fat: 9g
Saturated Fat: 1g
Cholesterol: 0mg
Sodium: 65mg
Total Carbohydrates: 29g
Dietary Fiber: 8g
Total Sugars: 18g
Protein: 6g

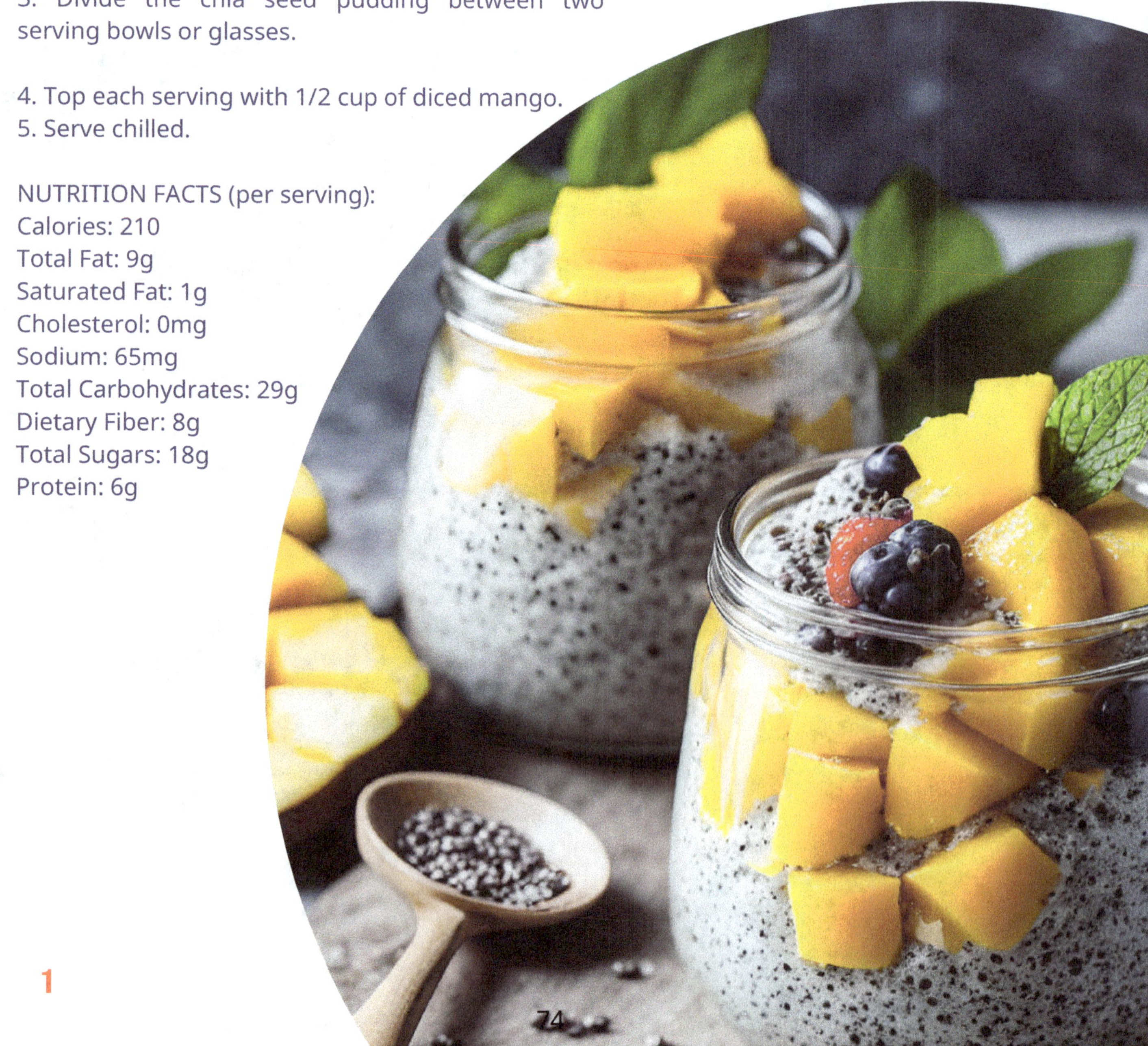

2. Dark Chocolate Avocado Mousse

Preparation Time: 10 minutes
Chilling Time: 2 hours
Total Time: 2 hours 10 minutes
Serves: 4

Ingredients:

 1 ripe avocado, pitted and peeled
- 1/4 cup unsweetened cocoa powder
- 1/4 cup maple syrup
- 1 teaspoon vanilla extract
- 1/4 teaspoon sea salt

Directions:

1. In a food processor or high-speed blender, combine the avocado, cocoa powder, maple syrup, vanilla extract, and sea salt. Blend until smooth and creamy, scraping down the sides as needed.

2. Transfer the mousse to a bowl or individual serving dishes. Cover and refrigerate for at least 2 hours, or until set.

3. Serve chilled.

NUTRITION FACTS (per serving):
Calories: 150
Total Fat: 10g
Saturated Fat: 2g
Cholesterol: 0mg
Sodium: 85mg
Total Carbohydrates: 16g
Dietary Fiber: 5g
Total Sugars: 9g
Protein: 3g

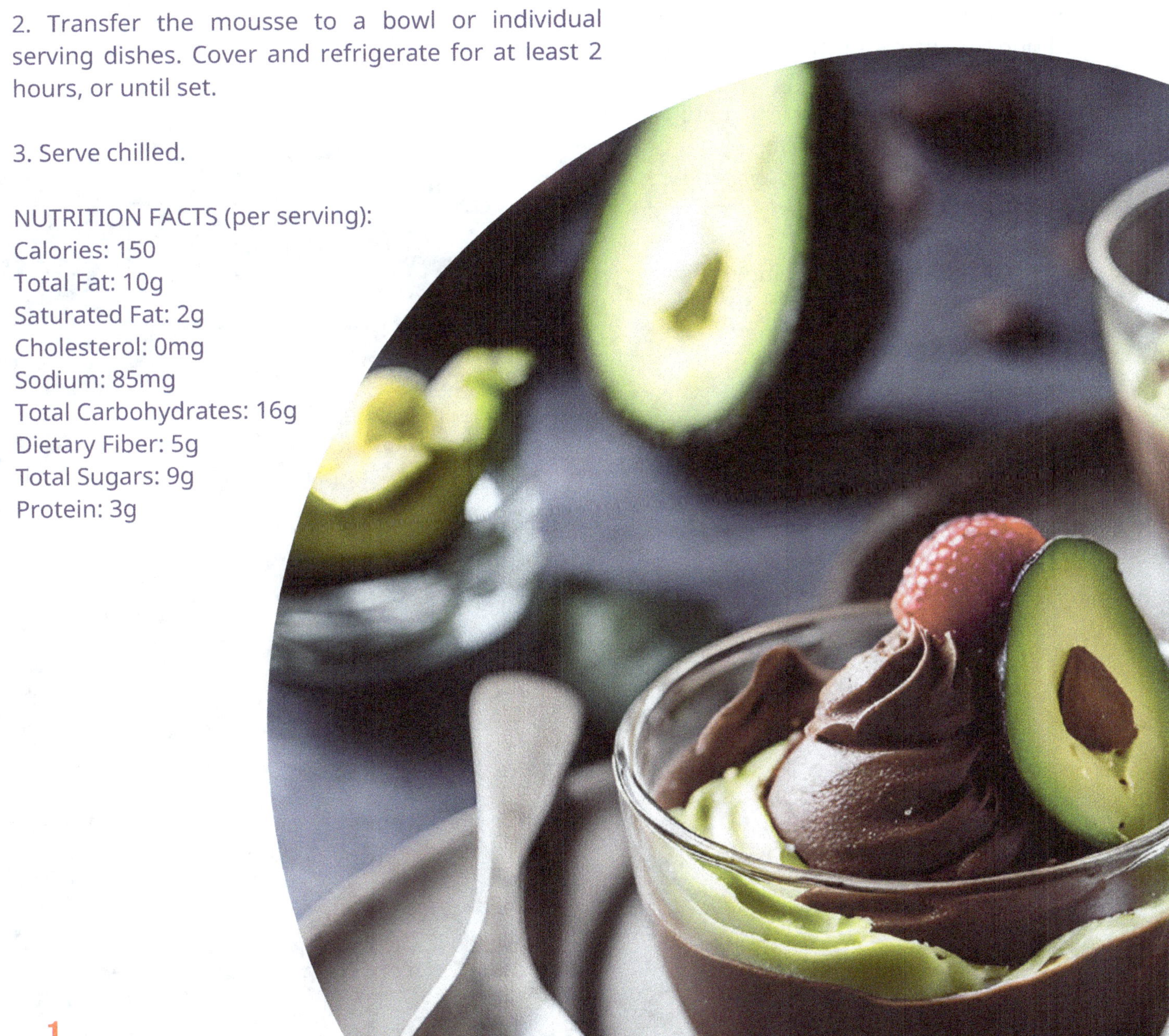

1

3. Baked Apples with Cinnamon

Preparation Time: 10 minutes
Cook Time: 30 minutes
Total Time: 40 minutes
Serves: 4

Directions:

1. Preheat the oven to 375°F.
2. Place the apple halves in a baking dish, cut-side up.
3. In a small bowl, mix together the brown sugar and cinnamon. Sprinkle the mixture evenly over the apple halves.
4. Pour the water into the baking dish around the apples.
5. Bake for 25-30 minutes, or until the apples are tender and the filling is bubbly.
6. Serve the baked apples warm, with a scoop of vanilla ice cream or whipped cream, if desired.

NUTRITION FACTS (per serving):
Calories: 100
Total Fat: 0g
Saturated Fat: 0g
Cholesterol: 0mg
Sodium: 0mg
Total Carbohydrates: 26g
Dietary Fiber: 4g
Total Sugars: 20g
Protein: 0g

Ingredients:

 4 medium apples, cored and halved
- 2 tablespoons brown sugar
- 1 teaspoon ground cinnamon
- 1/4 cup water
- Vanilla ice cream or whipped cream (optional)

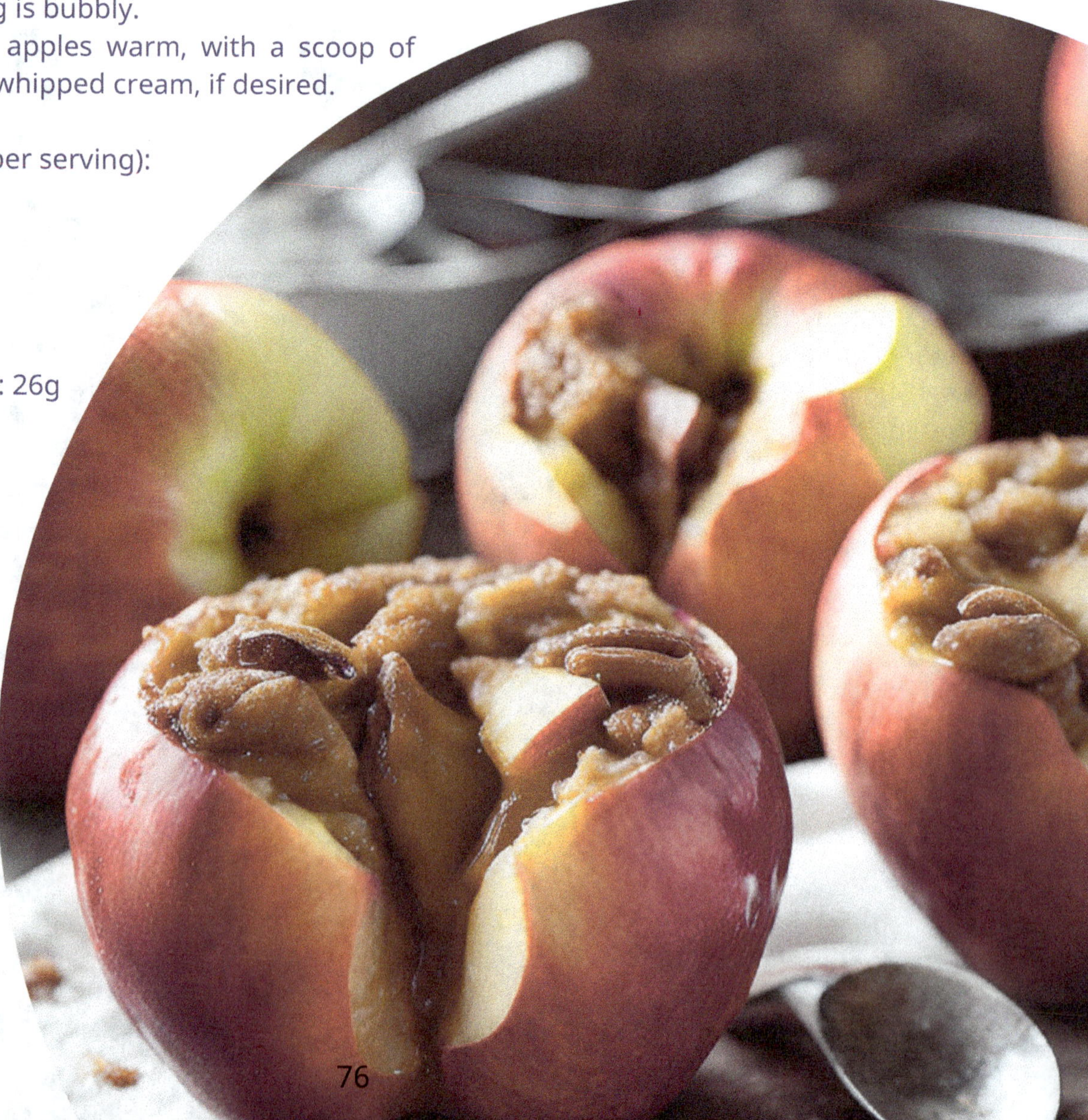

1

4. Berry Compote with Greek Yogurt

Preparation Time: 10 minutes
Cook Time: 15 minutes
Total Time: 25 minutes
Serves: 4

Ingredients:

2 cups mixed berries (such as blueberries, raspberries, and/or blackberries)
- 2 tablespoons honey
- 1 tablespoon lemon juice
- 1/4 teaspoon ground cinnamon
- 2 cups plain Greek yogurt

Directions:

1. In a small saucepan, combine the mixed berries, honey, lemon juice, and cinnamon.
2. Cook over medium heat, stirring occasionally, until the berries release their juices and the mixture thickens, about 15 minutes.
3. Remove from heat and let cool slightly.
4. Divide the Greek yogurt evenly among 4 serving bowls or glasses.
5. Top each serving of yogurt with a spoonful of the warm berry compote.
6. Serve immediately.

NUTRITION FACTS (per serving):
Calories: 150
Total Fat: 5g
Saturated Fat: 2g
Cholesterol: 10mg
Sodium: 45mg
Total Carbohydrates: 19g
Dietary Fiber: 3g
Total Sugars: 15g
Protein: 12g

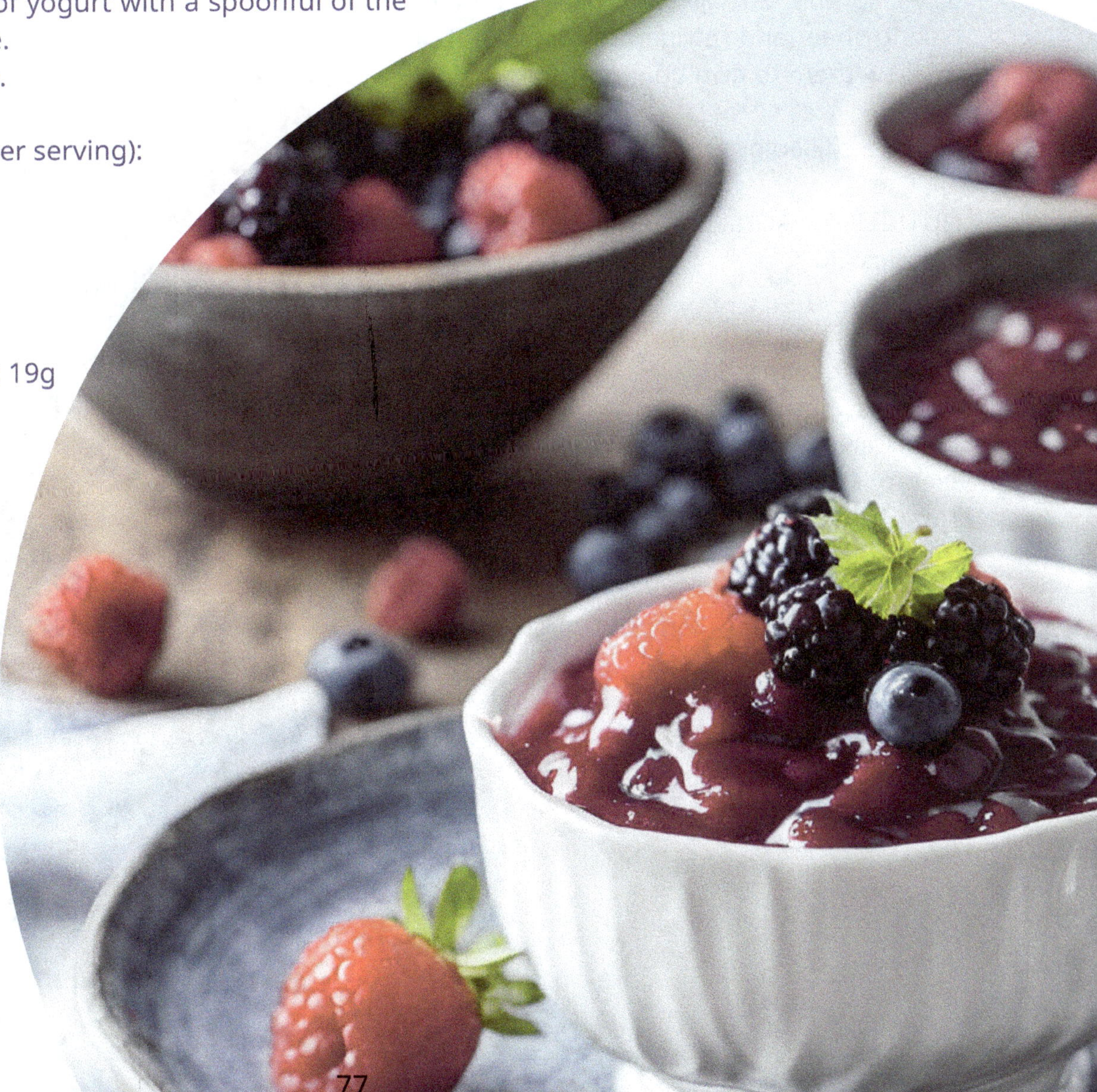

1

5. Pumpkin Spice Energy Balls

Preparation Time: 15 minutes
Chilling Time: 30 minutes
Total Time: 45 minutes
Serves: 12 (1 ball per serving)

Directions:

1. In a medium bowl, combine the rolled oats, pumpkin puree, almond butter, honey, pumpkin pie spice, cinnamon, and sea salt. Mix until well incorporated.

2. Using a small cookie scoop or your hands, form the mixture into 12 equal-sized balls.

3. Place the energy balls on a parchment-lined baking sheet and refrigerate for at least 30 minutes to allow them to firm up.

4. Serve chilled or at room temperature.

NUTRITION FACTS (per serving):
Calories: 90
Total Fat: 5g
Saturated Fat: 1g
Cholesterol: 0mg
Sodium: 55mg
Total Carbohydrates: 10g
Dietary Fiber: 2g
Total Sugars: 6g
Protein: 3g

Ingredients:

 1 cup rolled oats
- 1/2 cup pumpkin puree
- 1/4 cup almond butter
- 2 tablespoons honey
- 1 teaspoon pumpkin pie spice
- 1/4 teaspoon ground cinnamon
- 1/4 teaspoon sea salt

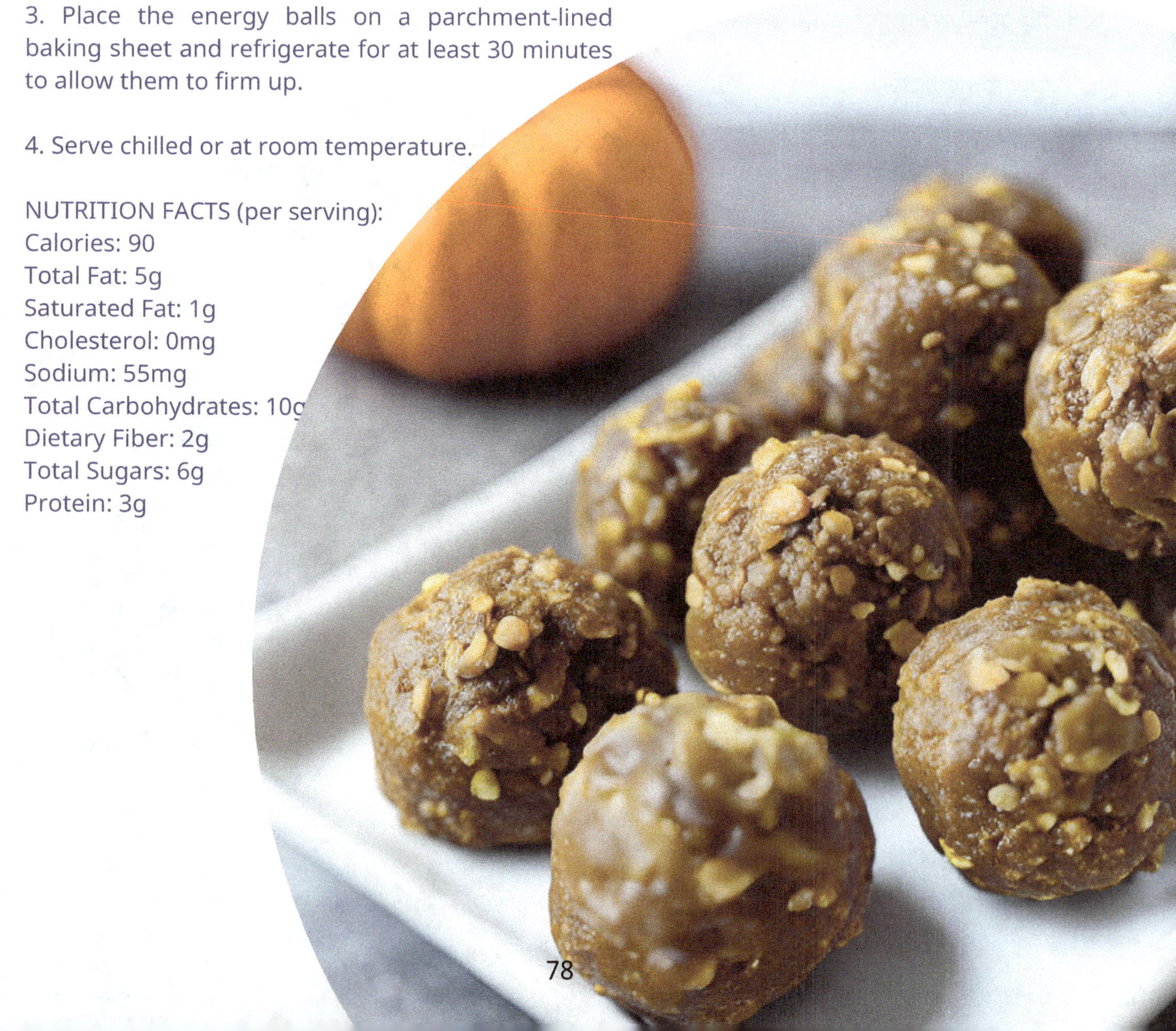

6. Banana and Almond Butter Ice Cream

Preparation Time: 10 minutes
Freezing Time: 4 hours
Total Time: 4 hours 10 minutes
Serves: 4

Ingredients:

 3 ripe bananas, peeled and frozen
- 2 tablespoons almond butter
- 1 tablespoon honey (optional)
- 1/4 teaspoon vanilla extract

Directions:

1. In a high-speed blender or food processor, combine the frozen bananas, almond butter, honey (if using), and vanilla extract.

2. Blend or process until smooth and creamy, scraping down the sides as needed.

3. Transfer the ice cream mixture to a freezer-safe container and freeze for at least 4 hours, or until firm.

4. Scoop and serve the banana almond butter ice cream.

NUTRITION FACTS (per serving):
Calories: 150
Total Fat: 7g
Saturated Fat: 1g
Cholesterol: 0mg
Sodium: 45mg
Total Carbohydrates: 21g
Dietary Fiber: 3g
Total Sugars: 14g
Protein: 3g

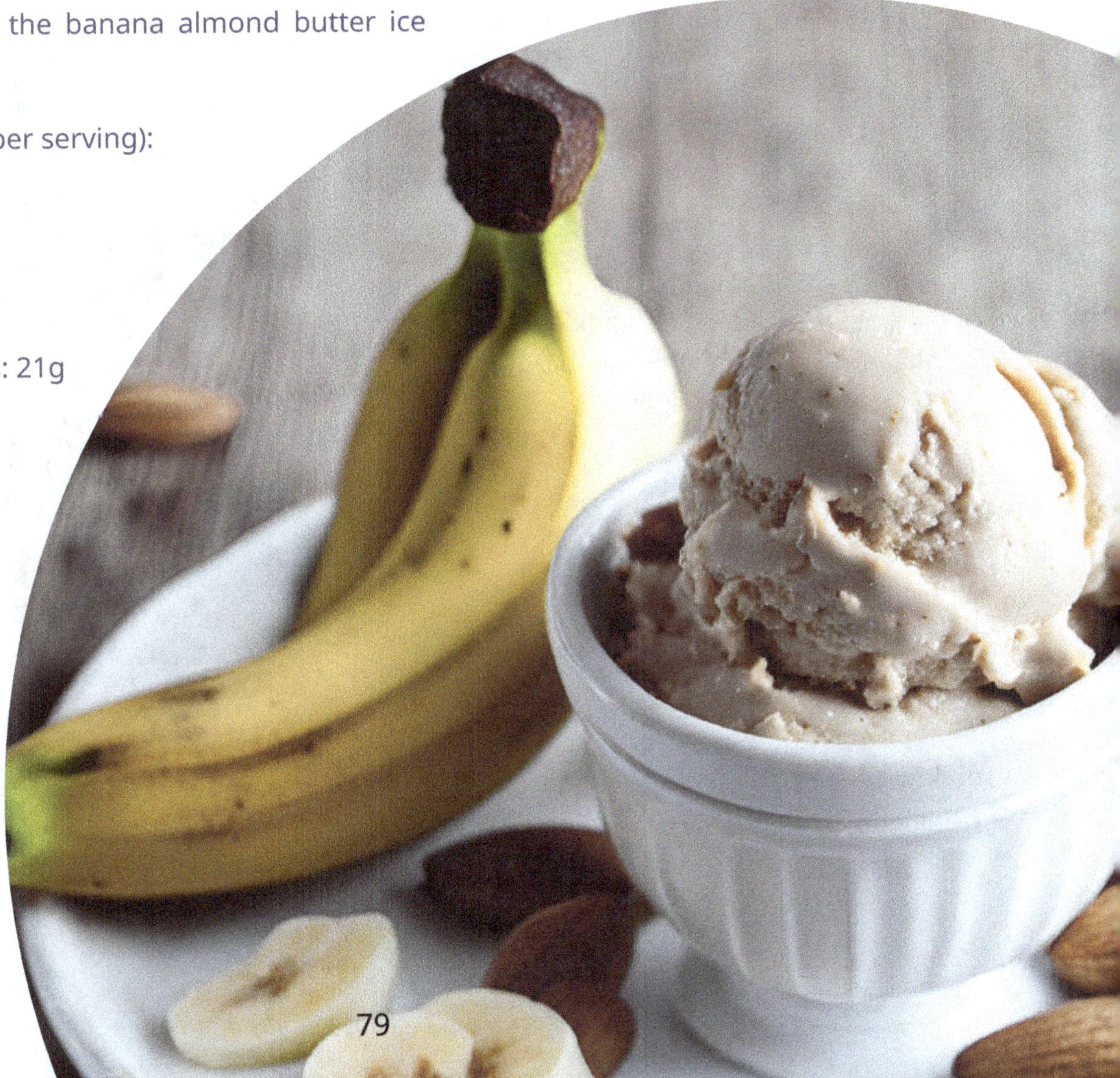

7. Oatmeal Raisin Cookies

Preparation Time: 15 minutes
Cook Time: 12 minutes
Total Time: 27 minutes
Serves: 18 cookies

Directions:

1. Preheat the oven to 350°F. Line two baking sheets with parchment paper.

2. In a large bowl, cream the butter and brown sugar together until light and fluffy, about 2-3 minutes. Beat in the egg and vanilla.

3. In a separate bowl, whisk together the flour, baking soda, cinnamon, and salt.

4. Gradually add the dry ingredients to the wet ingredients, mixing until just combined. Fold in the oats and raisins.

5. Scoop rounded tablespoons of dough onto the prepared baking sheets, spacing them about 2 inches apart.

6. Bake for 10-12 minutes, or until the edges are lightly golden. Allow the cookies to cool on the baking sheets for 5 minutes before transferring to a wire rack to cool completely.

NUTRITION FACTS (per cookie):
Calories: 170
Total Fat: 8g
Saturated Fat: 5g
Cholesterol: 25mg
Sodium: 105mg
Total Carbohydrates: 23g
Dietary Fiber: 2g
Total Sugars: 12g
Protein: 2g

Ingredients:

  1 cup (2 sticks) unsalted butter, softened
- 1 cup brown sugar
- 1 egg
- 1 teaspoon vanilla extract
- 1 1/2 cups all-purpose flour
- 1 teaspoon baking soda
- 1/2 teaspoon ground cinnamon
- 1/4 teaspoon salt
- 3 cups old-fashioned rolled oats
- 1 cup raisins

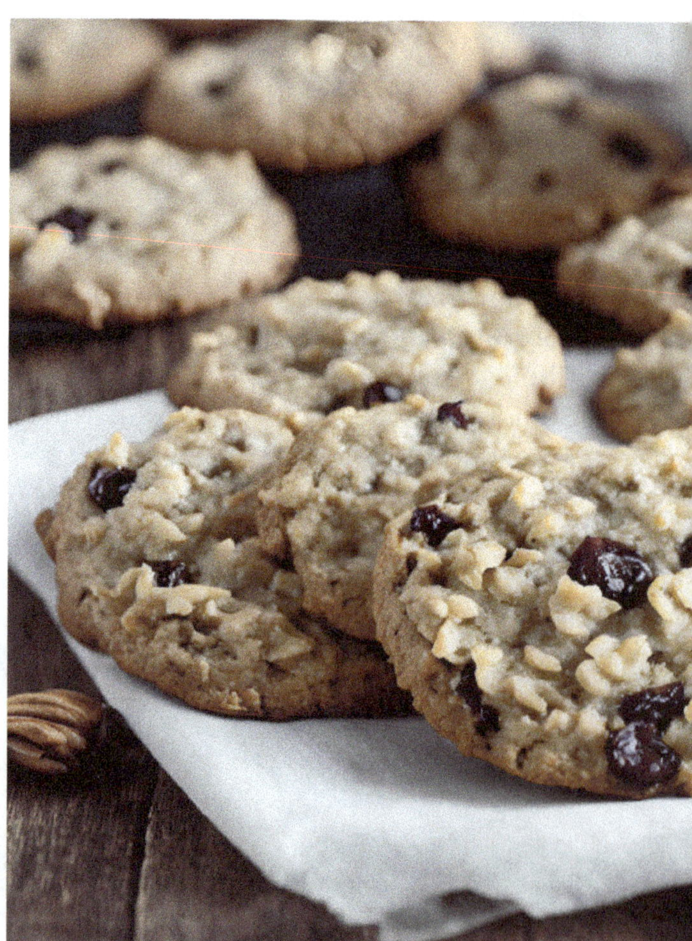

1

8. Coconut Macaroons

Preparation Time: 10 minutes
Cook Time: 15 minutes
Total Time: 25 minutes
Serves: 12 macaroons

Ingredients:

 2 large egg whites
- 1/3 cup granulated sugar
- 1/4 teaspoon salt
- 2 cups sweetened shredded coconut
- 1 teaspoon vanilla extract

Directions:

1. Preheat the oven to 325°F. Line a baking sheet with parchment paper.

2. In a medium bowl, beat the egg whites with an electric mixer until they are foamy. Gradually add the sugar and salt, beating until the mixture forms stiff, glossy peaks.

3. Gently fold in the shredded coconut and vanilla extract until well combined.

4. Scoop rounded tablespoons of the coconut mixture onto the prepared baking sheet, spacing them about 1 inch apart.

5. Bake for 12-15 minutes, or until the macaroons are lightly golden on the edges.

6. Remove the macaroons from the oven and let them cool on the baking sheet for 5 minutes before transferring to a wire rack to cool completely.

NUTRITION FACTS (per macaroon):
Calories: 90
Total Fat: 5g
Saturated Fat: 4g
Cholesterol: 0mg
Sodium: 55mg
Total Carbohydrates: 10g
Dietary Fiber: 1g
Total Sugars: 9g
Protein: 1g

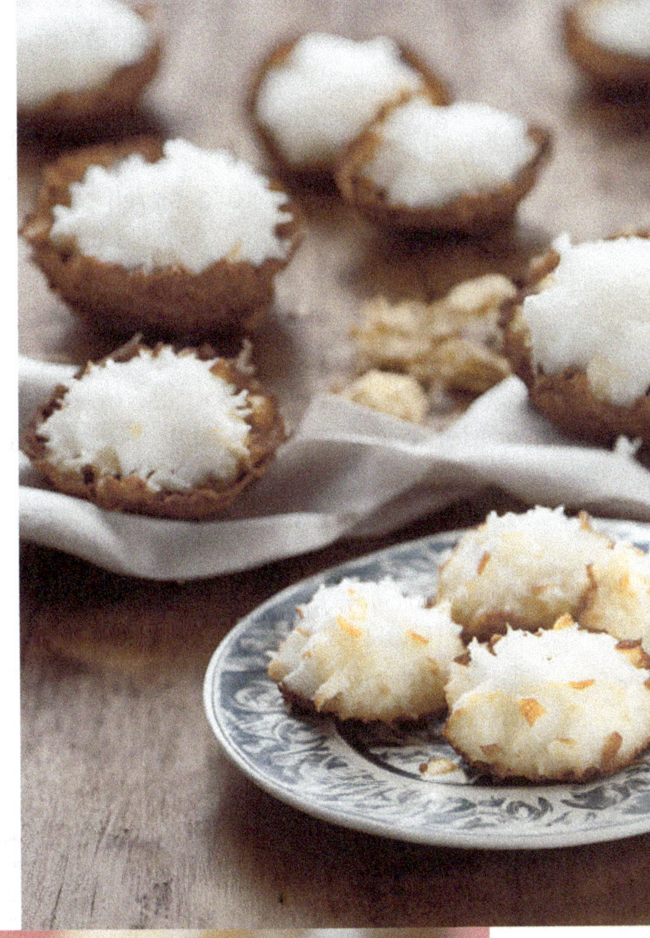

9. Berry and Almond Crisp

Preparation Time: 15 minutes
Cook Time: 30 minutes
Total Time: 45 minutes
Serves: 6

Ingredients:

For the Filling:
- 3 cups mixed berries (such as blueberries, raspberries, and/or blackberries)
- 2 tablespoons honey
- 1 tablespoon cornstarch
- 1 teaspoon lemon juice

For the Topping:
- 1 cup old-fashioned rolled oats
- 1/2 cup sliced almonds
- 1/4 cup whole wheat flour
- 2 tablespoons brown sugar
- 1/4 teaspoon ground cinnamon
- 4 tablespoons unsalted butter, melted

Directions:

1. Preheat the oven to 375°F. Grease a 9-inch baking dish.

2. In a medium bowl, combine the berries, honey, cornstarch, and lemon juice. Toss to coat the berries and transfer to the prepared baking dish.

3. In another bowl, mix together the oats, almonds, flour, brown sugar, and cinnamon. Stir in the melted butter until the mixture is well combined.

4. Sprinkle the oat topping evenly over the berry filling.

5. Bake for 25-30 minutes, or until the topping is golden brown and the filling is bubbly.

6. Allow the crisp to cool for 10 minutes before serving.

NUTRITION FACTS (per serving):
Calories: 260
Total Fat: 12g
Saturated Fat: 4g
Cholesterol: 15mg
Sodium: 10mg
Total Carbohydrates: 35g
Dietary Fiber: 5g
Total Sugars: 16g
Protein: 5g

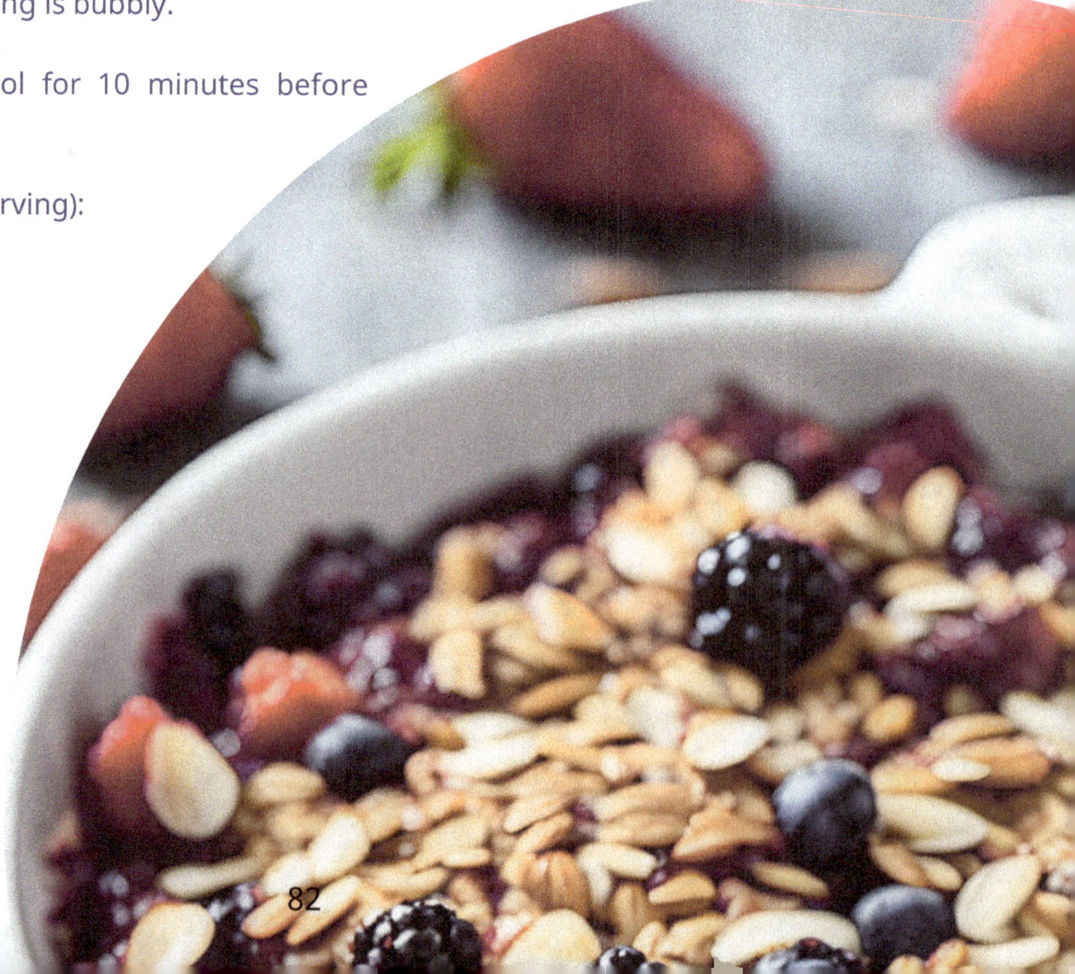

10. Chocolate Chia Pudding

Preparation Time: 10 minutes
Chilling Time: 4 hours
Total Time: 4 hours 10 minutes
Serves: 4

Directions:

1. In a medium bowl, whisk together the chia seeds, almond milk, cocoa powder, maple syrup, vanilla extract, cinnamon, and salt until well combined.

2. Cover the bowl and refrigerate for at least 4 hours, or overnight, stirring occasionally, until the mixture has thickened to a pudding-like consistency.

3. Divide the chocolate chia pudding into 4 serving bowls or glasses.

4. Top with your desired toppings, such as sliced strawberries, toasted coconut flakes, or chopped nuts.
5. Serve chilled.

NUTRITION FACTS (per serving):
Calories: 160
Total Fat: 7g
Saturated Fat: 1g
Cholesterol: 0mg
Sodium: 65mg
Total Carbohydrates: 22g
Dietary Fiber: 8g
Total Sugars: 9g
Protein: 5g

Ingredients:

1/4 cup chia seeds
- 2 cups unsweetened almond milk
- 1/4 cup unsweetened cocoa powder
- 2 tablespoons maple syrup
- 1 teaspoon vanilla extract
- 1/4 teaspoon ground cinnamon
- Pinch of salt

Toppings (optional):
- Sliced strawberries
- Toasted coconut flakes
- Chopped nuts

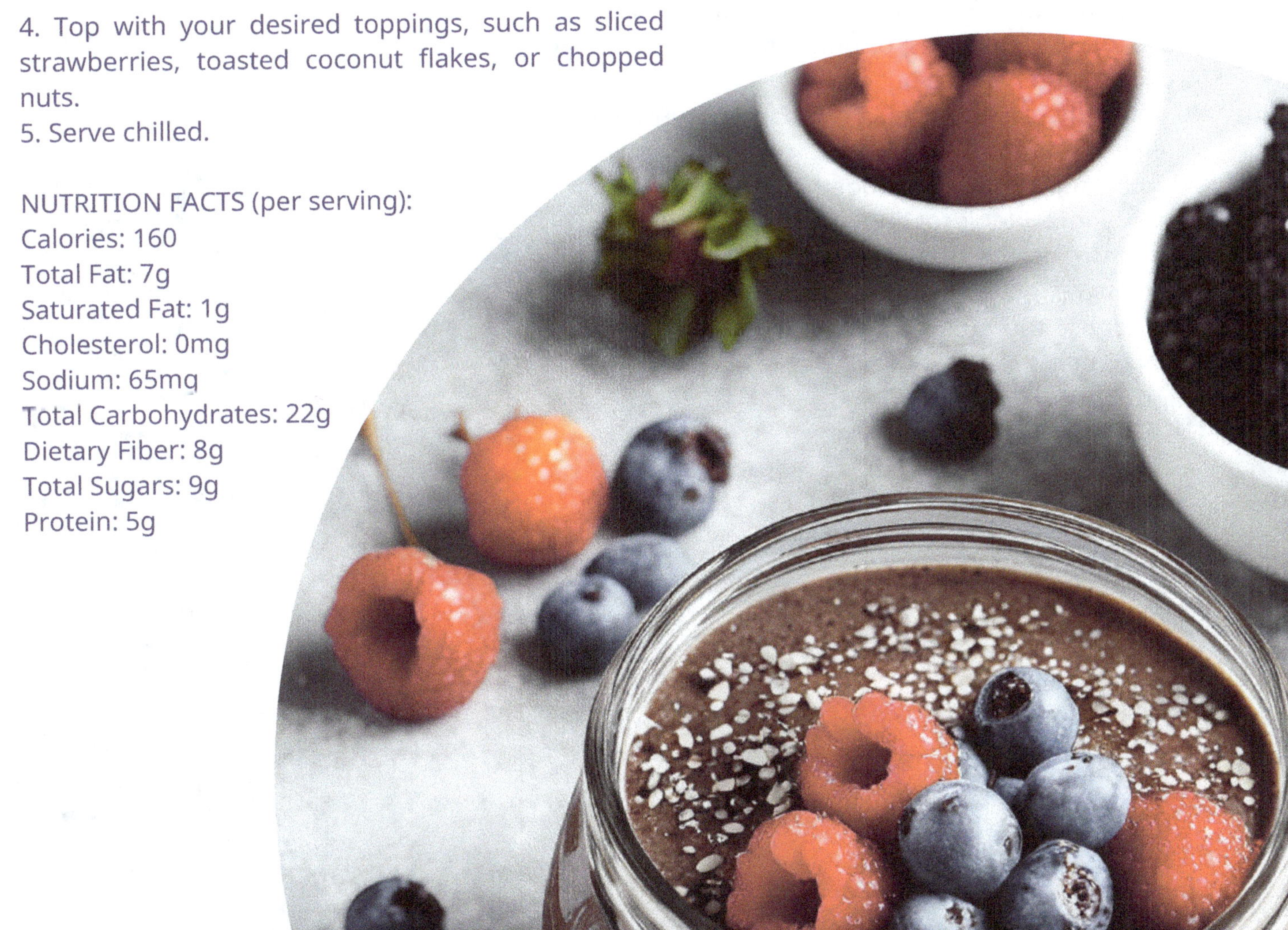

11. Lemon Yogurt Cake

Preparation Time: 15 minutes
Cook Time: 40 minutes
Total Time: 55 minutes
Serves: 8

Directions:

1. Preheat the oven to 350°F. Grease a 9-inch round baking pan and line the bottom with parchment paper.
2. In a medium bowl, whisk together the flour, baking powder, and salt.
3. In a large bowl, beat the yogurt and granulated sugar until well combined. Beat in the eggs one at a time, then stir in the lemon zest and vegetable oil.
4. Gradually fold the dry ingredients into the wet ingredients until just combined, being careful not to overmix.
5. Pour the batter into the prepared baking pan and bake for 35-40 minutes, or until a toothpick inserted into the center comes out clean.
6. Allow the cake to cool in the pan for 10 minutes, then invert it onto a wire rack to cool completely.
7. In a small bowl, whisk together the confectioners' sugar and 2-3 tablespoons of lemon juice to make a glaze. Drizzle the glaze over the top of the cooled cake.
8. Serve the lemon yogurt cake at room temperature.

NUTRITION FACTS (per serving):
Calories: 290
Total Fat: 9g
Saturated Fat: 1g
Cholesterol: 65mg
Sodium: 190mg
Total Carbohydrates: 47g
Dietary Fiber: 1g
Total Sugars: 32g
Protein: 6g

Ingredients:

 1 1/2 cups all-purpose flour
- 2 teaspoons baking powder
- 1/4 teaspoon salt
- 1 cup plain Greek yogurt
- 1 cup granulated sugar
- 3 large eggs
- 2 tablespoons grated lemon zest (about 2 lemons)
- 1/3 cup vegetable oil
- 2 tablespoons freshly squeezed lemon juice

For the Glaze:
- 1 cup confectioners' sugar
- 2-3 tablespoons freshly squeezed lemon juice

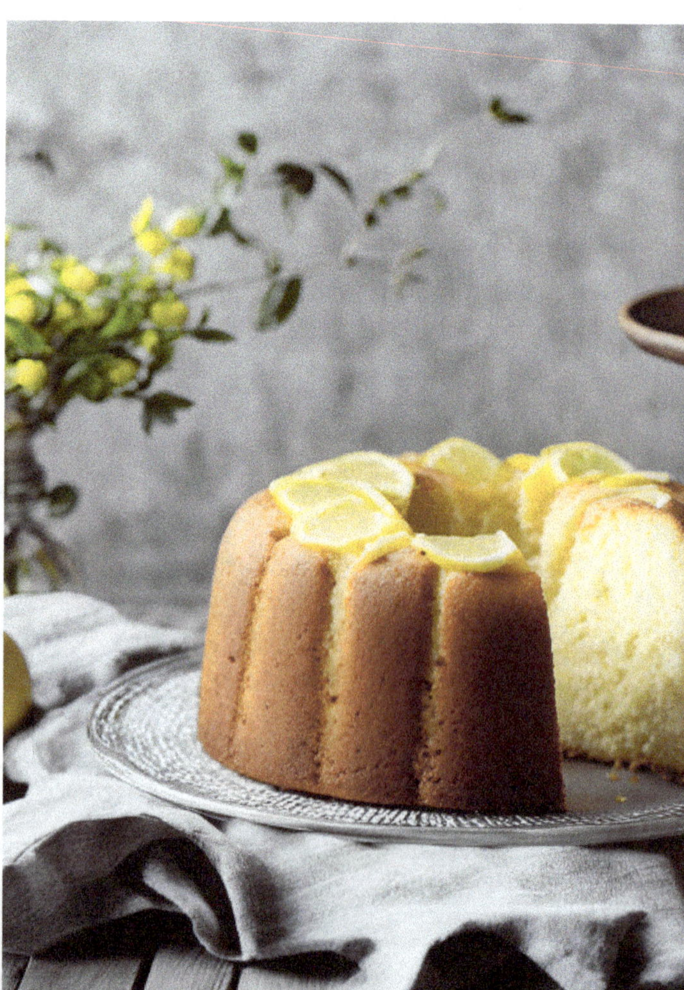

12. Fruit Salad with Mint

Preparation Time: 15 minutes
Chilling Time: 30 minutes
Total Time: 45 minutes
Serves: 4

Ingredients:

 1 cup diced pineapple
- 1 cup diced mango
- 1 cup halved strawberries
- 1 cup blueberries
- 2 tablespoons freshly squeezed orange juice
- 1 tablespoon honey
- 2 tablespoons chopped fresh mint leaves

Directions:

1. In a large bowl, combine the diced pineapple, mango, strawberries, and blueberries.

2. In a small bowl, whisk together the orange juice and honey.

3. Pour the orange juice mixture over the fruit and gently toss to coat.

4. Sprinkle the chopped mint leaves over the fruit salad.

5. Cover and refrigerate for at least 30 minutes to allow the flavors to meld.
6. Serve chilled.

NUTRITION FACTS (per serving):
Calories: 120
Total Fat: 0g
Saturated Fat: 0g
Cholesterol: 0mg
Sodium: 0mg
Total Carbohydrates: 30g
Dietary Fiber: 4g
Total Sugars: 24g
Protein: 1g

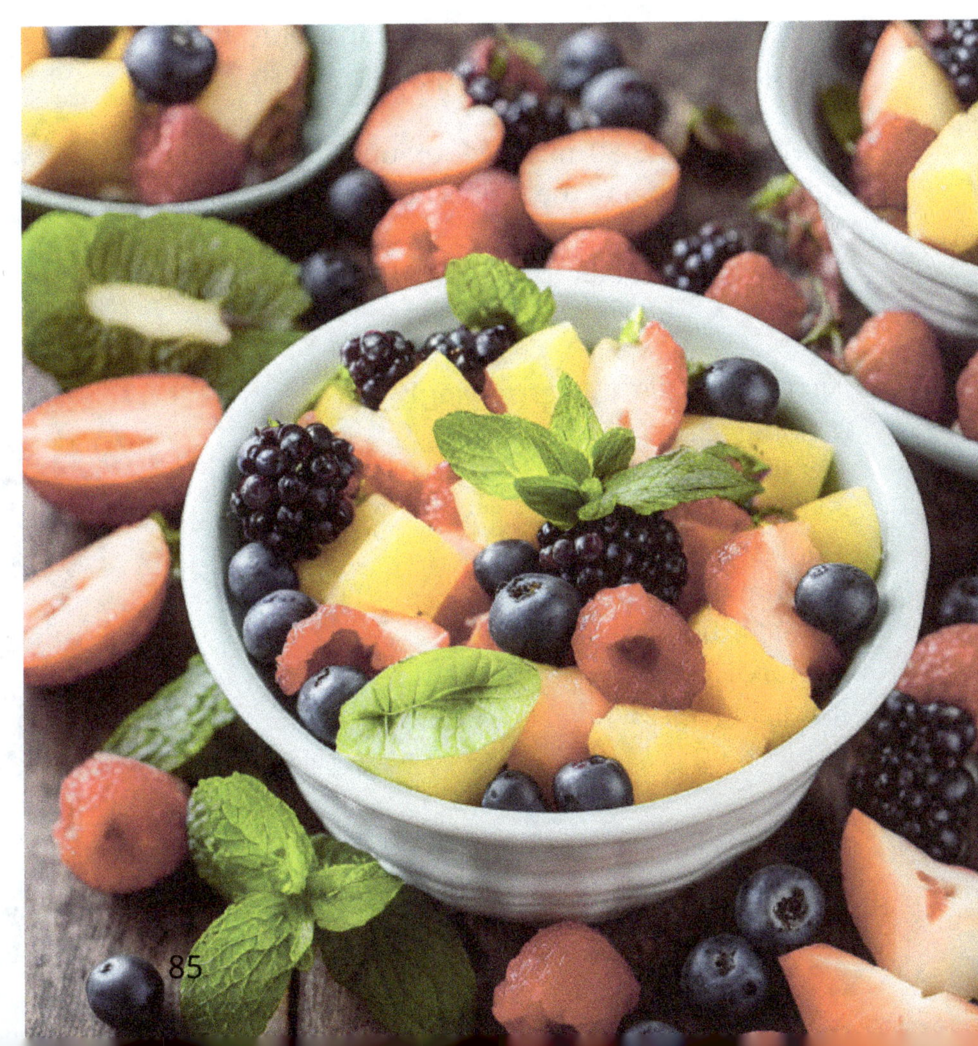

13. Peach and Blueberry Cobbler

Preparation Time: 20 minutes
Cook Time: 30 minutes
Total Time: 50 minutes
Serves: 6

Directions:

1. Preheat the oven to 375°F. Grease a 9-inch baking dish.

2. In a large bowl, combine the sliced peaches, blueberries, 1/4 cup sugar, cornstarch, and lemon juice. Toss to coat the fruit and transfer to the prepared baking dish.

3. In a medium bowl, whisk together the flour, 1/4 cup sugar, baking powder, and salt. Cut in the cold butter using a pastry blender or two forks until the mixture resembles coarse crumbs. Stir in the milk until just combined.

4. Drop the batter by large spoonfuls onto the fruit filling, spreading it to the edges of the dish.

5. Bake for 25-30 minutes, or until the topping is golden brown and the fruit is bubbly.

6. Allow the cobbler to cool for 10-15 minutes before serving.

NUTRITION FACTS (per serving):
Calories: 290
Total Fat: 10g
Saturated Fat: 6g
Cholesterol: 25mg
Sodium: 260mg
Total Carbohydrates: 47g
Dietary Fiber: 3g
Total Sugars: 26g
Protein: 4g

Ingredients:

For the Filling:
- 3 cups sliced fresh peaches (about 4-5 medium peaches)
- 2 cups fresh blueberries
- 1/4 cup granulated sugar
- 1 tablespoon cornstarch
- 1 teaspoon lemon juice

For the Topping:
- 1 cup all-purpose flour
- 1/4 cup granulated sugar
- 2 teaspoons baking powder
- 1/4 teaspoon salt
- 5 tablespoons cold unsalted butter, cubed
- 1/2 cup milk

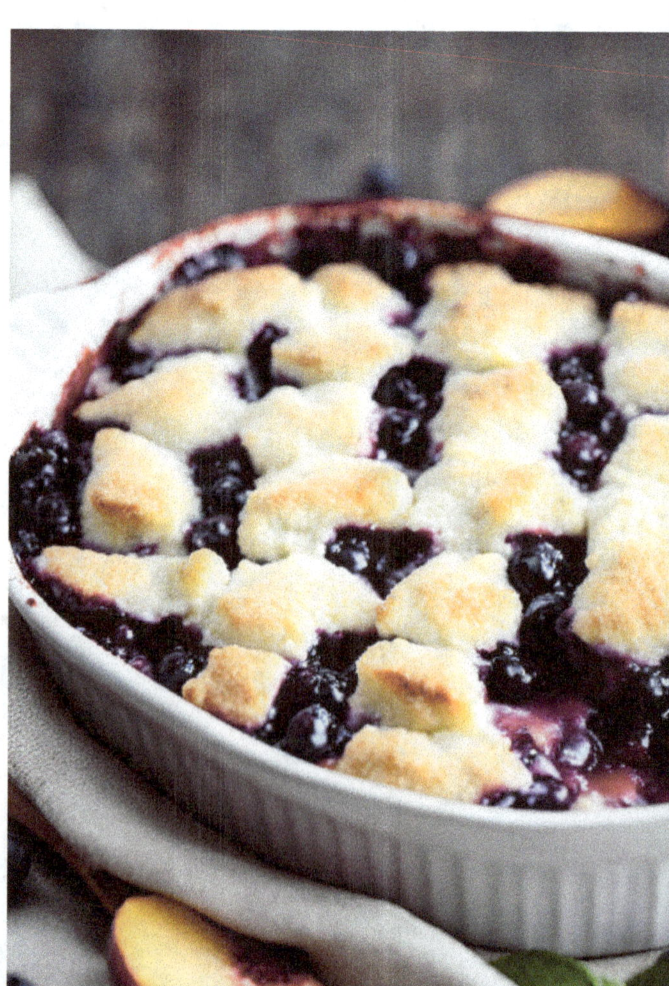

Chapter 10 : Managing Weight Gain during Menopause.

Weight gain during menopause is a common concern for many women. The hormonal changes that occur during this time can make it more challenging to maintain a healthy weight. Decreased estrogen levels, slower metabolism, and changes in body composition all contribute to this issue. However, with mindful eating, regular physical activity, and strategic dietary choices, it is possible to manage weight effectively during menopause.

Understanding the Causes of Weight Gain

- **Hormonal Changes:** The drop in estrogen levels during menopause can lead to increased fat storage, particularly around the abdomen. Estrogen helps regulate body weight by influencing glucose and lipid metabolism. When estrogen levels decline, the body tends to store more fat.

- **Slower Metabolism:** As we age, our metabolic rate naturally slows down. This means that our bodies require fewer calories to function, making it easier to gain weight if we continue to eat the same amount of food as we did in our younger years.

- **Loss of Muscle Mass:** Age-related muscle loss, known as sarcopenia, reduces the number of calories the body burns at rest. Muscle tissue burns more calories than fat tissue, so maintaining muscle mass is crucial for a healthy metabolism.

- **Lifestyle Factors:** Sedentary lifestyles, poor dietary choices, and stress can all contribute to weight gain during menopause. Many women find that they are less active than they were in their younger years, which can further exacerbate weight gain.

Strategies for Managing Weight Gain

- **Balanced Diet:** Focus on a balanced diet that includes a variety of nutrient-dense foods. This helps ensure that your body gets the vitamins and minerals it needs while managing calorie intake.

- **Portion Control:** Be mindful of portion sizes to avoid overeating. Eating smaller, more frequent meals can help control hunger and prevent overeating.

- **Regular Physical Activity:** Incorporate both cardiovascular exercises and strength training into your routine. Cardio exercises, such as walking, jogging, or swimming, help burn calories, while strength training helps build and maintain muscle mass.

- **Healthy Snacks:** Opt for healthy snacks that are high in protein and fiber to keep you feeling full and satisfied. Avoid sugary and processed snacks that can lead to weight gain.

- **Stay Hydrated:** Drink plenty of water throughout the day. Sometimes, thirst can be mistaken for hunger, leading to unnecessary snacking.

- **Limit Sugar and Refined Carbs:** Reduce your intake of sugary foods and refined carbohydrates, which can lead to weight gain and increased blood sugar levels.

- ***Manage Stress:*** Practice stress-reducing activities such as yoga, meditation, or deep breathing exercises. Stress can lead to emotional eating and weight gain.

- ***Get Enough Sleep:*** Ensure you get 7-9 hours of quality sleep each night. Poor sleep can disrupt hormones that regulate hunger and appetite, leading to weight gain.

Managing weight gain during menopause involves a combination of healthy eating, regular physical activity, and lifestyle changes. By focusing on nutrient-dense foods, maintaining muscle mass through strength training, and practicing mindful eating, you can effectively manage your weight and support your overall health during this significant life transition. The recipes provided in this chapter are designed to help you stay on track with your weight management goals while enjoying delicious, satisfying meals.

Chapter 11 : Boosting Mood and Energy through Food

Menopause brings about various physiological and psychological changes that can significantly affect mood and energy levels. Fluctuating hormone levels, particularly the decrease in estrogen, can lead to symptoms such as fatigue, irritability, anxiety, and depression. While these symptoms are common, they can be managed effectively through a balanced diet that supports both mental and physical well-being.

Understanding the Link Between Diet and Mood

- **Hormonal Balance:** Certain foods can help stabilize hormones and reduce mood swings. For example, phytoestrogens found in soy products can help balance estrogen levels.

- **Blood Sugar Levels:** Maintaining stable blood sugar levels is crucial for preventing energy dips and mood swings. Eating regular meals and snacks that combine protein, healthy fats, and complex carbohydrates can help keep blood sugar levels steady.

- **Brain Function:** Nutrients such as omega-3 fatty acids, B vitamins, and antioxidants are essential for brain health and can improve mood and cognitive function.

- **Inflammation:** Chronic inflammation is linked to depression and fatigue. Anti-inflammatory foods, such as fruits, vegetables, nuts, seeds, and fatty fish, can help reduce inflammation and improve overall mood.

Key Nutrients for Boosting Mood and Energy

- **Omega-3 Fatty Acids:** Found in fatty fish (salmon, mackerel, sardines), flaxseeds, chia seeds, and walnuts. Omega-3s are essential for brain health and can help reduce symptoms of depression and anxiety.

- **B Vitamins:** Important for energy production and brain function. Sources include whole grains, legumes, eggs, dairy products, and leafy greens.

- **Magnesium:** Helps regulate neurotransmitters and can improve sleep and reduce anxiety. Found in nuts, seeds, whole grains, and leafy green vegetables.

- **Antioxidants:** Protect brain cells from oxidative stress and improve overall cognitive function. Abundant in berries, dark chocolate, nuts, and colorful fruits and vegetables.

- **Protein:** Essential for maintaining muscle mass and energy levels. Sources include lean meats, poultry, fish, eggs, dairy products, legumes, and tofu.

Chapter 12 : Addressing Common Menopausal Symptoms with Diet

Menopause can bring about a wide range of symptoms due to hormonal changes in the body. These symptoms can include hot flashes, night sweats, mood swings, sleep disturbances, and more. While these symptoms are a natural part of the menopausal transition, they can often be managed or alleviated through dietary adjustments. This chapter explores how specific foods and nutrients can help address common menopausal symptoms and improve overall well-being.

Hot Flashes and Night Sweats

Hot flashes and night sweats are among the most common and uncomfortable symptoms of menopause. They can disrupt sleep and significantly impact quality of life. Certain foods and dietary practices can help manage these symptoms:

- *Phytoestrogens:* These plant compounds mimic estrogen in the body and can help balance hormone levels. Good sources include soy products (tofu, tempeh, soy milk), flaxseeds, sesame seeds, and whole grains.

- *Hydration:* Staying well-hydrated can help regulate body temperature. Drink plenty of water throughout the day and include hydrating foods such as cucumbers, watermelon, and leafy greens.

- *Avoid Triggers:* Spicy foods, caffeine, and alcohol can trigger hot flashes for some women. Keeping a food diary can help identify and avoid personal triggers.

Mood Swings and Irritability

Hormonal fluctuations during menopause can lead to mood swings and irritability. Nutritional strategies can help stabilize mood and improve mental well-being:

- *Omega-3 Fatty Acids:* These healthy fats support brain health and can help reduce symptoms of depression and anxiety. Good sources include fatty fish (salmon, mackerel, sardines), flaxseeds, chia seeds, and walnuts.

- *B Vitamins:* Essential for energy production and brain function, B vitamins can help improve mood. Sources include whole grains, legumes, eggs, dairy products, and leafy greens.

- *Complex Carbohydrates:* These help maintain steady blood sugar levels, which can stabilize mood. Opt for whole grains, oats, sweet potatoes, and legumes.

Sleep Disturbances

Sleep disturbances are another common issue during menopause, often exacerbated by hot flashes and night sweats. Certain foods and nutrients can promote better sleep:

- *Magnesium:* This mineral helps relax muscles and calm the nervous system, promoting better sleep. Sources include nuts, seeds, whole grains, and leafy green vegetables.

- *Tryptophan:* An amino acid that helps produce serotonin and melatonin, both of which are important for sleep. Found in turkey, chicken, eggs, nuts, and seeds.

- *Herbal Teas:* Teas such as chamomile, valerian root, and lavender can have a calming effect and promote sleep.

Bone Health

As estrogen levels decline, women are at a higher risk for osteoporosis and bone fractures. Adequate intake of calcium and vitamin D is crucial for maintaining bone health:

- *Calcium:* Essential for strong bones, calcium can be found in dairy products, leafy green vegetables, tofu, and fortified foods.

- *Vitamin D:* Helps the body absorb calcium. Sources include fatty fish, fortified dairy products, and exposure to sunlight.

- *Magnesium and Vitamin K:* These nutrients also support bone health. Magnesium is found in nuts, seeds, and whole grains, while vitamin K is abundant in leafy green vegetables.

Digestive Issues

Menopause can also bring about digestive issues such as bloating, gas, and changes in bowel habits. A diet rich in fiber and probiotics can help maintain a healthy digestive system:

- *Fiber:* Promotes healthy digestion and regular bowel movements. Sources include fruits, vegetables, whole grains, and legumes.

- *Probiotics:* Beneficial bacteria that support gut health. Found in yogurt, kefir, sauerkraut, kimchi, and other fermented foods.

- *Hydration:* Drinking plenty of water aids in digestion and prevents constipation.

By incorporating these nutrient-rich foods and recipes into your diet, you can effectively manage common menopausal symptoms and support your overall health. Adjusting your diet to include specific nutrients can help address hot flashes, mood swings, sleep disturbances, bone health, and digestive issues, making the transition through menopause smoother and more manageable.

Chapter 13 : Planning and Preparing Your Meals for Success.

Planning and preparing meals is a crucial aspect of maintaining a healthy diet, especially during menopause. With the right strategies, you can ensure that you are consuming balanced, nutritious meals that support your overall well-being and help manage menopausal symptoms. This chapter provides practical tips and strategies for effective meal planning and preparation, along with some easy-to-follow recipes.

Benefits of Meal Planning

- **Nutritional Balance:** Planning your meals in advance ensures that you include a variety of nutrient-dense foods, helping you meet your dietary needs.

- **Time Efficiency:** Preparing meals ahead of time saves you from last-minute cooking stress, making it easier to stick to healthy eating habits.

- **Cost-Effective:** Buying ingredients in bulk and reducing food waste can save money.

- **Portion Control:** Preparing meals ahead allows you to control portion sizes, which is important for managing weight.

Steps to Successful Meal Planning

- **Assess Your Nutritional Needs:** Consider your dietary requirements, focusing on foods that alleviate menopausal symptoms and support overall health. Include plenty of fruits, vegetables, whole grains, lean proteins, and healthy fats.

- **Create a Weekly Menu:** Plan your meals for the week, including breakfast, lunch, dinner, and snacks. Make sure to incorporate a variety of foods to keep your meals interesting and nutritionally balanced.

- **Make a Shopping List:** Based on your weekly menu, create a detailed shopping list. Stick to the list to avoid impulse purchases and ensure you have all necessary ingredients.

- **Prep in Advance:** Set aside time to prep ingredients or cook meals in advance. This could include chopping vegetables, cooking grains, or preparing complete meals that can be reheated during the week.

- **Utilize Storage Solutions:** Invest in quality storage containers to keep your prepped food fresh. Label containers with dates to keep track of freshness.

Tips for Meal Preparation

- *Batch Cooking:* Cook large batches of grains, proteins, and vegetables that can be mixed and matched throughout the week.

- *Freezer-Friendly Meals:* Prepare meals that can be frozen and reheated for convenience. Soups, stews, and casseroles are great options.

- *One-Pot Meals:* Simplify cooking and cleanup by making one-pot meals like stir-fries, sheet-pan dinners, and slow-cooker recipes.

- *Healthy Snacks:* Prepare healthy snacks such as cut-up vegetables, fruit, nuts, and yogurt to have on hand for quick, nutritious options.

Sample Meal Plan

Monday
- Breakfast: Greek yogurt with mixed berries and honey

- Lunch: Quinoa and black bean salad with avocado and lime dressing

- Dinner: Baked salmon with roasted asparagus and sweet potatoes

- Snack: Apple slices with almond butter

Tuesday
- Breakfast: Overnight oats with chia seeds and banana

- Lunch: Grilled chicken and vegetable wrap

- Dinner: Lentil soup with a side of mixed greens salad

- Snack: Carrot sticks with hummus

Wednesday
- Breakfast: Smoothie with spinach, avocado, berries, and almond milk

- Lunch: Tofu and vegetable stir-fry with brown rice

- Dinner: Turkey chili with cornbread

- Snack: Greek yogurt with walnuts and honey

Thursday
- Breakfast: Scrambled eggs with spinach and whole grain toast

- Lunch: Tuna salad with mixed greens and olive oil dressing

- Dinner: Stuffed bell peppers with quinoa and black beans

- Snack: Fresh fruit salad

Friday
- Breakfast: Cottage cheese with pineapple and chia seeds

- Lunch: Chickpea and vegetable curry with brown rice

- Dinner: Grilled shrimp with zucchini noodles and pesto

- Snack: Handful of mixed nuts

Saturday
- Breakfast: Whole grain pancakes with fresh berries and maple syrup

- Lunch: Turkey and avocado sandwich on whole grain bread

- Dinner: Baked cod with roasted Brussels sprouts and quinoa

- Snack: Dark chocolate squares

Sunday
- Breakfast: Smoothie bowl with granola, banana, and blueberries

- Lunch: Lentil and vegetable soup with a side of whole grain bread

- Dinner: Grilled chicken with a side of roasted root vegetables

- Snack: Celery sticks with peanut butter

Planning and preparing meals for success during menopause involves thoughtful consideration of your nutritional needs and practical strategies to make healthy eating easy and sustainable. By taking the time to plan your meals, shop smartly, and prepare ingredients in advance, you can ensure that you are nourishing your body with the foods it needs to thrive during this stage of life. The recipes provided offer a delicious and varied way to incorporate essential nutrients into your diet, helping to manage menopausal symptoms and support overall health.

Conclusion

As you navigate the transformative journey of menopause, the importance of a thoughtful and nourishing diet cannot be overstated. The transition through menopause can bring about a host of changes—physically, emotionally, and mentally. By making informed dietary choices, you can significantly influence how your body copes with these changes, improving your overall well-being and quality of life.

Recap of Key Points

1. Understanding Menopause: Recognizing the stages of menopause and their impact on the body is crucial. Each stage presents unique challenges that can be mitigated through tailored nutritional strategies.

2. The Role of Nutrition: A balanced diet rich in essential nutrients can help manage menopausal symptoms such as hot flashes, mood swings, weight gain, and sleep disturbances. Specific nutrients like phytoestrogens, omega-3 fatty acids, calcium, and magnesium play pivotal roles in alleviating these symptoms.

3. Meal Planning and Preparation: Effective meal planning and preparation are vital for maintaining a healthy diet. By organizing your meals and preparing ingredients in advance, you can ensure that you consistently consume balanced, nutrient-dense foods.

4. Delicious Recipes: The variety of recipes provided in this book offers practical, tasty options that incorporate key nutrients necessary for managing menopausal symptoms. These recipes are designed to be easy to prepare and adaptable to individual tastes and dietary needs.

Empowerment through Knowledge

Empowerment comes from knowledge and understanding. By educating yourself about the nutritional needs specific to menopause and making conscious choices about what you eat, you take control of your health and well-being. This proactive approach can help you navigate menopause with greater ease and confidence.

Final Thoughts

As you implement the dietary strategies and recipes provided in this book, take note of the positive changes in your body and mind. Celebrate your progress, no matter how small, and continue to explore new ways to nourish yourself.

Your journey through menopause is a testament to your strength and resilience. With the right tools and knowledge, you can make this transition a time of renewal and empowerment. Here's to a healthy, happy, and vibrant menopausal journey!